Charting the Experience of Children and Adolescents Affected by Emotional Neglect

This timely and compelling volume explores the interdisciplinary perspectives on, and long-term consequences of, emotional neglect on children and adolescents, creating a theoretical model that considers the impact of emotional neglect in distinct phases of development.

Paying specific attention to Bronfenbrenner's ecological systems theory which hypothesised that a child's development is impacted by their interactions with different systems within their environment, this book takes a unique and chronological look at neglect. Starting from prenatal development up to early adulthood, its chapters underpin research through exploration of other theories such as attachment theory, cognitive development theory, social learning theory and emotional schema to highlight the importance of recognising the negative consequences of emotional neglect, and encourage the development of interventions that support healthy emotional development in children.

This book will appeal to scholars, researchers and postgraduate students working in child and family social work, child abuse and neglect research, as well as child and adolescent psychiatry and clinical psychology. Practitioners working with children and adolescents may also find this volume informative and useful.

Ewa Wojtyna is Doctor of Psychology, cognitive-behavioural therapist and a medical doctor, Institute of Medical Science, University of Opole, Poland.

Marcin Gierczyk is Doctor of Social Sciences in Pedagogy, associate professor, University of Silesia in Katowice, Poland.

The Mental Health and Well-being of Children
and Adolescents
Series Editor: Garry Hornby (University of Plymouth)

Mental health disorders in children and young people are increasing, with one in four under-16s experiencing mental health difficulties which will disrupt relationships, education and work. In addition to this, one in ten under-16s suffers from a diagnosed disorder. Access to up-to-date research and appropriate interventions minimises the mental health challenges these children and adolescents face and reduces their potentially lifelong impact.

It has been internationally recognised that the scale of mental health research is low in relation to the burden of the disorder. This research-focused series will consist of titles that consider key issues affecting young people's mental health and well-being, exploring preventative measures, promoting positive behaviour, and sharing research to develop effective and efficient treatment.

Aimed primarily at researchers and postgraduate students, this series will also be of interest to practitioners in the mental health field, such as psychologists, and some in the field of education, such as counsellors, who would like to implement research-based findings in their clinical practice.
Books in the series include:

Mental Health and Quality of Life of Adolescents with Physical, Intellectual and Developmental Disabilities
Perspectives of Parents and Children
Zenon Gajdzica, Stanisława Byra, Anna Kołodziej-Zaleska, Katarzyna Rutkowska and Daniela Dzienniak-Pulina

Promoting Children's Mental Health and Well Being
Importance of Partnerships in Building Resilient and Empathic Children
Rebecca P. Ang

Charting the Experience of Children and Adolescents Affected by Emotional Neglect
Ewa Wojtyna and Marcin Gierczyk

Please visit www.routledge.com/The-Mental-Health-and-Well-being-of-Children-and-Adolescents/book-series/MHWCA.

Charting the Experience of Children and Adolescents Affected by Emotional Neglect

Ewa Wojtyna and Marcin Gierczyk

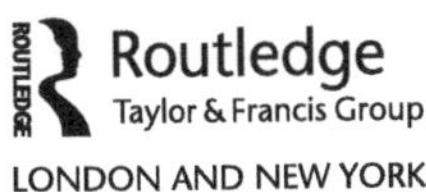

LONDON AND NEW YORK

First published 2025
by Routledge
4 Park Square, Milton Park, Abingdon, Oxon OX14 4RN

and by Routledge
605 Third Avenue, New York, NY 10158

Routledge is an imprint of the Taylor & Francis Group, an informa business

British Library Cataloguing-in-Publication Data
A catalogue record for this book is available from the British Library

ISBN: 9781032616728 (hbk)
ISBN: 9781032621180 (pbk)
ISBN: 9781032621203 (ebk)

DOI: 10.4324/9781032621203

Typeset in Sabon
by codeMantra

To all those who have suffered in silence

Contents

About the authors

Ewa Wojtyna, MD, PhD

Ewa Wojtyna is Doctor of Psychology, cognitive-behavioural therapist and a medical doctor at the Institute of Medical Sciences at the University of Opole. She is psychiatrist, psychologist, cognitive-behavioural therapist and supervisor. Her research interests include the psychosocial determinants of human mental and somatic health. As a psychotherapist, he focuses on working with complex trauma, the consequences of emotional neglect and psychosomatic problems. She is interested in changes in the modern world and their impact on human development and quality of life.

Marcin Gierczyk, PhD

Marcin Gierczyk is Doctor of Social Sciences in Pedagogy, associate professor at the Institute of Pedagogy of the University of Silesia in Katowice, Poland. He is a Crisis Intervention specialist focusing on domestic violence and child protection. He has gained valuable academic knowledge from institutions such as the University of Birmingham, the University of Erlangen-Nuremberg, the University of Oxford and the University of Oslo. Associate member of the McGill Centre for Research on Children and Families (CRCF) in Canada and an Honorary Research Fellow at the Jubilee Centre for Character and Virtues, School of Education, the University of Birmingham (UK). His research interests include the environmental and educational support of gifted children and youth, emotional neglect, domestic violence, child protection and methodological solutions for diagnosing and optimising the well-being of children and adolescents.

Series editor introduction

It is now over 20 years since the need for an increased focus on child and adolescent mental health and well-being, particularly in schools, was highlighted by the publication of the first of several books on the topic (Atkinson & Hornby, 2002). This handbook provides information on a wide range of child and adolescent mental health issues and concerns. It focuses on the identification and treatment of mental health problems and disorders, which are even more relevant today in our post-pandemic world in which stresses on families and children are continually increasing. One response to the publication of this handbook has been the creation of a series of books which is dedicated to addressing the mental health and well-being of children and adolescents. The key focus of books in this series is on evaluating the latest theory and research available and disseminating evidence-based interventions and programmes. This book is the eighth in the series.

The first book in the series addressed the issue of bullying in schools (Cowie & Myers, 2018), while the second book examined various approaches for promoting the mental health of children in schools (Reupert, 2020). The third book focused specifically on the use of mindfulness meditation for facilitating the mental health and well-being of children and young people in schools and community settings (Singh & Singh Joy, 2021). The fourth book addressed bullying in schools from multiple perspectives (Rigby, 2022), and the fifth book focused on implications for children's mental health of the Covid-19 pandemic (Kauffman & Badar, 2023). The sixth book presented findings from a research study of health-related quality of life of three groups of adolescents, those with physical disability, intellectual disability and foetal alcohol spectrum disorder (Gajdzica et al., 2024). The seventh book provided a timely scholarly and practical evaluation of the critical imperative of enhancing children's mental health and well-being in our 21st-century world (Ang, 2024).

The current book makes an important original contribution to the series, as it focuses on an area that has been under-researched in the field of children's mental health and well-being, that is emotional neglect. The first chapter discusses the definition of 'neglect' and its subtypes. Four different theoretical models of the phenomenon are presented: the parental deficit model, the ecological deficit model, the ecological-transactional model and ecological systems theory. The second chapter discusses how modern health paradigms, like the biomedical and biopsychosocial models, are now seen as less adequate due to their inability to encapsulate the complex and rapidly evolving nature of contemporary health issues. The third chapter discusses how social behaviour is associated with complex neurobiological processes and how neglect in close relationships leads to chronic stress and mental and somatic health problems, including depressive disorders and other neuropsychiatric problems. The fourth chapter describes the mechanisms of emotional development in infancy, considering the child-parent relationship and potential emotional neglect. Developmental manifestations and consequences of neglecting children are presented, starting from newborns and ending with children one year old. The fifth chapter explores the crucial period of toddlerhood, focusing on the rapid brain development that occurs during these years. It examines the significance of social interactions in emotional growth and the distinction between appropriate nurturing and excessive concern for children's development. The sixth chapter focuses on children aged three to six years and the key elements involved in supporting their harmonious development, highlighting the role of parents and caregivers in shaping their social and emotional skills. The seventh chapter addresses the main developmental milestones of middle childhood when children begin to form strong relationships with their peers and their education becomes increasingly important. The eighth chapter focuses on the roles of parents and social systems, that is schools, peers and the virtual environment, in adolescent development at ages 12 to 18 years. It explores the consequences of neglect, highlighting autonomy, self-identity and the quest for uniqueness and gender identity construction. It provides an overview of how neglect influences the adolescent experience and shapes developmental trajectories. The ninth chapter presents the findings of empirical research on emotional neglect to explore how neglect experienced in childhood affects self-perception and emotional functioning in adulthood. The final chapter proposes a model for understanding emotional neglect and its consequences, including contemporary socio-cultural phenomena, such as breaking the vicious circle related to striving for maximum child development and primarily focusing on correcting deficits in children and adolescents. Effective therapy methods to address the effects of emotional neglect are discussed. Finally, it is concluded that protecting children from the effects of emotional neglect is crucial in preventing mental health disorders in children and adolescents, and reducing potential consequences such as self-harm, suicide and death.

Emeritus Professor Garry Hornby,
University of Plymouth, June 2024

Preface

There were many reasons to write this book. First, childhood should be a period in a person's life where positive experiences such as feeling safe and carefree, having fun and being loved should dominate. It is a time when children develop emotionally, socially and intellectually. A sense of security is the foundation that allows a child to explore the world and learn through playing freely. The love from family members creates a stable emotional background, which is essential for developing self-esteem. Second, the reality is that childhood is not always idyllic, and there exist many phenomena that can profoundly disrupt the positive growth of children and young people. One of these phenomena is emotional neglect, a social problem which cannot be ignored because of its long-term consequences for both children and adolescents. Therefore, its far-reaching effects are analysed in this book.

The focus of this book is on systematising knowledge in the field of neglect, particularly in the field of human growth, starting from infant development, through to early adulthood, and creating a theoretical model which takes into account the influence of emotional neglect in distinct phases of development. Until recently it has been impossible to build a single model describing basic mechanisms characteristic of this phenomenon, which makes it difficult to properly diagnose and as a consequence apply appropriate forms of intervention. The aim of this book is to address this by considering research and theories concerning the various aspects and features of neglect. Because of the significance of neglect at various stages of development, the effects of neglect are viewed differently for children and adolescents, taking into consideration the different developmental needs for both these age groups. Therefore, parental behaviour is viewed differently, depending on whether the neglect is of the needs of younger children or adolescents.

It should be emphasised that emotional neglect is not the same as emotional abuse. Emotional abuse involves doing things that can be emotionally hurtful, while emotional neglect means not doing something that improves the emotional well-being of children and adolescents (Kumari, 2020). It is also worth noting that in contemporary discourse on child emotional neglect, it is increasingly emphasised that it is not just a matter of passive indifference on the part of parents. In fact, emotional neglect can also have an active dimension. Although involved, parents may focus on realising their own ideas and scenarios about what is best for their child rather than actually responding to their child's emotional needs. This approach may stem from parents' deeply held beliefs about what constitutes "child wellbeing", often stemming from their own experiences, aspirations or fears. As a result, although parents may be actively involved in their child's life, their actions do not necessarily support the child's emotional development in the way that the child needs. In practice, this means that parents may impose on the child the different activities, educational or social pathways they think are best without considering the child's real interests, needs and emotions. This can lead to a misunderstanding and lack of emotional support on the part of parents, possibly resulting in emotional and developmental problems. Therefore, parents need to be aware of this subtle but significant difference and try to really listen to their children's needs and not just impose their own beliefs about what is best for them.

It is essential to bear in mind that the understanding of emotional neglect is influenced by the cultural context and social norms relating to parenting and the role of the carer. It is worth noting that what is considered the norm in one society may not be acceptable in another. Social norms influence an individual's thoughts and behaviour (Schultz et al., 2007; Klika et al., 2019) and legal acts. For example, there are still countries where corporal punishment is not fully prohibited, e.g. Arabia, Singapore, Dominica, Barbados and India.

Scientifically, the issue of emotional neglect has been highlighted relatively recently, since the 1950s, although the problems associated with children's emotional neglect were observed much earlier. Initially, the problem was not analysed as a separate category in child well-being research, and research mainly focused on physical neglect or abuse, ignoring the subtler forms of neglect that have long-lasting effects on the emotional and psychological development of children and young people.

As child psychology and psychiatry have progressed, more attention has begun to be paid to the impact of the home environment and parental interactions on children's emotional health. It has been realised that emotional neglect, i.e. a lack of adequate attention, support and sensitivity to a child's emotional needs, leads to serious mental health problems such as, but not limited to, depression, anxiety, relationship problems or difficulties in emotional self-regulation, which generates significant social costs. Research focusing on emotional neglect has more recently contributed to the development of new therapeutic and intervention methods to prevent its adverse effects. Today, emotional neglect is treated as an important risk factor in the development of psychopathology, and its recognition and therapy have become key elements of modern psychological and psychotherapeutic care.

This is the first book to focus on the stages of life development from infancy through adolescence to investigate what we currently know from interdisciplinary perspectives about emotional neglect, with regard to multiple mental health challenges. We decided to structure this book chronologically through different life stages, since available data indicates that emotional neglect of children should be considered distinct from the neglect of adolescents, as there are differences in the needs of these age groups. Parents' behaviours are also distinct and different across life stages, which poses different threats to children and adolescents (Jankowiak, 2019).

Ewa Wojtyna & Marcin Gierczyk
Katowice, June 2024

Acknowledgements

We would like to thank the reviewers of this book, who are valued experts in the field of child abuse: Professors Christine Wekerle from McMaster University (Canada), Delphine Collin-Vézina from McGill University (Canada), M. Catherine Maternowska from the University of Edinburgh (United Kingdom) and Rebecca Ang Pei-Hui from Nanyang Technological University (Singapore).

Chapter 1

Emotional neglect

A problem that has been neglected for too long

Emotional neglect – in comparison to other forms of abuse – is a topic that has long been overshadowed in discussions of child and adolescent mental health, particularly from a theoretical perspective. This is highlighted by Ylitervo et al. (2023, p. 1), emphasising that in the context of emotional neglect, "there is a lack of research on its prevalence in the general population". These authors refer to meta-analyses to confirm this (e.g. Stoltenborgh et al., 2013, p. 352), where only 13 articles on emotional neglect, including 59,655 participants, were identified between 1980 and 2008. In contrast, Mathews et al. (2020) identified 23 articles between the years 2005 and 2019. The reason for this can be attributed to the fact that the negative consequences of emotional neglect are seen with more of a delay than is the case with other forms or subtypes of neglect. It is important to note that emotional neglect is one of the more subtle but simultaneously devastating forms of inadequate parental care, which can have a profound impact on a child's social, emotional and cognitive development (Glaser, 2002; Young et al., 2011). Emotional neglect is a central concern of the present book, in which we adopt, like Prior and Quinn (2010), the definition described by Erickson and Egeland (2002, p. 14) to be, "passive or passive-aggressive inattention to the child's emotional needs, nurturing, or emotional well-being" performed by "psychologically unavailable parents who overlook their children's cues for warmth and comfort".

Emotional neglect is widespread (Gilbert et al., 2009; Keyes et al., 2012), as studies in developed countries have found that the prevalence of emotional neglect is 18.4% (Stoltenborgh et al., 2013, 2015). The effects of neglect on a child's development can be at least as harmful as the consequences of physical or sexual abuse (Hildyard & Wolfe, 2002; Schimmenti et al., 2015). This is an important finding, as physical and sexual abuse are often seen as the forms of maltreatment with the most significant negative impact (Musetti et al., 2016).

Neglect

Before considering the phenomenon of emotional neglect from different perspectives, it is first necessary to define the concept of "neglect" and its

DOI: 10.4324/9781032621203-1

subtypes. Definitions of "neglect" are a key element in the scientific discourse on child abuse or maltreatment, reflecting the diversity of approaches and perspectives in the field. The specificity of the definition of neglect depends on the conception of neglect we adopt – whether we see it as a homogenous phenomenon or use typology to distinguish its different forms. This distinction is fundamental to research, diagnosis and intervention, as it allows for a more precise identification of intervention and educational needs. Rebbe (2018, p. 304) points out that, in the literature, "there is a lack of consensus on what constitutes neglect or how it should be defined". This is related to what Dubowitz et al. (1993, 2004) point out, that neglect is a heterogeneous phenomenon in terms of the behaviours and situational factors that comprise it. There is additionally a cultural understanding and identification of child neglect (Baker, 2009). As can be seen, definitions of neglect vary in their detail. Two examples of general definitions of neglect are presented below:

> Neglect is a condition in which a caretaker responsible for the child, either deliberately or by extraordinary inattentiveness, permits the child to experience avoidable present suffering and/or fails to provide one or more of the ingredients generally deemed essential for developing a person's physical, intellectual, and emotional capacities.
>
> (Polansky et al., 1981, p. 15)

> Neglect occurs when the basic needs of children are not met, regardless of cause. 'Basic needs' include adequate shelter, food, health care, clothing, education, protection and nurturance.
>
> (Dubowitz et al., 1993, p. 12)

We consider that the two definitions complement each other, offering a broad view of child neglect, while each emphasises slightly different aspects of the phenomenon. The former may be more useful in the context of therapeutic and educational work, focusing on the effects of neglect on child development. Whereas, the latter may be more relevant in the planning and implementing of social and material interventions to meet children's basic needs. Experts in the field of child neglect, in an attempt to deal with the lack of unanimity as to the definition and categories of neglect, have developed a division of children's experiences into broader subtypes (see Table 1.1).

Each categorisation reflects the different authors' perspectives on child neglect, highlighting the common, as well as the different, aspects they consider most prevalent. This diversity of categories highlights the complexity of the concept of neglect and its diverse impacts on children's development and well-being.

Table 1.1 Categories of neglect representing different authors' views

Category	Definition	Main effects	Behaviour examples	Diagnosis and intervention	Immediate protection indicated
Physical neglect Dubowitz et al. (2004), Slack et al. (2003), Kaufman Kantor et al. (2004), Erickson and Egeland (2002)	Lack of basic physical needs and a safe environment.	Growth disorders, malnutrition, chronic diseases.	Not providing adequate food, clothing, hygiene.	Verification of living conditions, consultations with a dietitian, regular health check-ups.	Yes
Mental health neglect Slack et al. (2003), Erickson and Egeland (2002), Brassard and Donovan (2006), Trickett et al. (2009)	Ignoring emotional and psychological needs, lack of emotional support.	Emotional problems, depression, anxiety.	Not responding to the child's emotional needs, ignoring warning signs of mental health issues.	Psychological assessment of the child, therapy, emotional support for the child and family.	Yes
Cognitive neglect Slack et al. (2003), Kaufman Kantor et al. (2004)	Neglect of educational and developmental needs, lack of intellectual stimulation.	Developmental delays, learning difficulties, low self-esteem.	Not providing access to education, lack of interest in school progress.	Developmental assessment, educational support, therapies to support intellectual development.	Rarely
Supervision neglect Kaufman Kantor et al. (2004)	Insufficient supervision of the child, allowing dangerous behaviours.	Accidents, injuries, involvement in criminal activity.	Allowing dangerous play, lack of supervision in potentially dangerous situations.	Assessment of family situation, education of caregivers on safety, institutional supervision if necessary.	Usually

(Continued)

Table 1.1 (Continued)

Category	Definition	Main effects	Behaviour examples	Diagnosis and intervention	Immediate protection indicated
Medical neglect Erickson and Egeland (2002)	Not providing necessary medical care, ignoring health problems.	Worsening health condition, chronic diseases, death.	Ignoring medical advice, not providing medications, delaying doctor visits.	Medical assessment of the child, ensuring access to healthcare, legal intervention if necessary.	Yes
Environmental neglect Dubowitz et al. (2004)	Failure to provide a safe and appropriate environment, including exposure to harmful elements.	Increased risk of injury, health problems due to unsanitary conditions, psychological distress.	Exposing the child hazardous conditions, lack of safe living space, allowing the child to live in unsanitary conditions.	Environmental assessment, immediate intervention to improve living conditions, collaboration with housing and social services.	Usually
Education neglect Erickson and Egeland (2002)	Educational neglect, not ensuring access to education and proper support in learning.	Low education, difficulties in finding a job, low self-esteem.	Not enrolling the child in school, ignoring the compulsory education duty, lack of support in home learning.	Assessment of the child's educational situation, cooperation with educational institutions, providing educational support.	Rarely

Emotional neglect

Emotional neglect is a form of neglect that includes a lack of appropriate emotional response, caregiver unavailability and lack of interaction between the caregiver and the child (Ban & Oh, 2016; Cicchetti & Toth, 2005; Glaser, 2002). It refers to the failure to meet the child's emotional needs such as support, affection and providing the child with a sense of love (Dube et al., 2003). It is a condition in which a child's emotional needs are ignored or inadequately met, with serious consequences for the child's mental and emotional development. Emotional neglect is recognised as a major risk factor for psychopathology, meaning that it increases the likelihood of various psychiatric disorders (Jin et al., 2023; Young et al., 2011), problems related to self-image, emotion regulation and self-esteem (Colvert et al., 2008), which promotes the development of depression and anxiety. In the field of psychology and healthcare, understanding emotional neglect as a factor affecting mental health is crucial. Wark et al. (2003, p. 1034) note that, "despite the lack of a clear definition of emotional neglect, there is a general consensus that emotional neglect is related to the attachment or formation of a cohesive bond between a child and his/her parents". Hayashi (2022), on the other hand, highlights the complexity and challenges of defining emotional neglect, which is one form of child abuse and neglect.

It is impossible to analyse emotional neglect in isolation from other forms of abuse. Whereas empirical evidence does not support the assumption that emotional and physical neglect are more likely to co-occur than other types of abuse (Grummitt et al., 2022), it should be noted that those who experienced emotional neglect were more likely to experience physical neglect compared to those who did not experience emotional neglect (Dong et al., 2004).

In analysing the phenomenon of emotional neglect, it is crucial to consider two basic premises. The first relates to the co-occurrence of emotional and physical neglect, suggesting that it is difficult to separate their individual effects. The second is that both types of neglect have similar effects on the development of mental health (Infurna et al., 2016). Jin et al. (2023, p. 2) disagree with this, emphasising that "emotional and physical neglect are distinct experiences". As Grummitt et al. (2022, p. 1) pointed out, "research that combines emotional and physical neglect into a single exposure may obscure relationships with mental health". Studies by Grummitt et al. (2022), Lee et al. (2018), and Salokangas et al. (2020), noted that emotional neglect significantly predicted depression, anxiety, substance abuse and stress, whereas physical neglect did not. Aust et al. (2013) investigated the relationship between early emotional neglect and alexithymia, a personality trait characterised by difficulties in identifying and expressing personal feelings, which is known to be a risk factor for affective disorders. A study of a non-clinical sample of individuals with high and low levels of alexithymia found a significant positive correlation between alexithymia and early emotional neglect, suggesting that it may predict overall levels of alexithymia. Whereas, this correlation was not observed for sexual abuse and physical neglect.

There is no theory that fully explains why emotional neglect of children happens. Four different causal models or theories of emotional neglect are presented: the parental deficit model, the ecological deficit model, the ecological-transactional model (Valtolina et al., 2023) and ecological systems theory (Bronfenbrenner, 1989). Each of these models offers a different perspective on the reasons, emphasising the multifaceted nature of emotional neglect. Analysing the definitions of emotional neglect, we can see that these models overlap, providing a broad perspective for understanding the reasons for the different subtypes of neglect.

The parental deficit model (Cameron et al., 2007) identifies the parents with their mental health conditions and their characteristics as the cause of child neglect. For example, parents may lack the necessary parenting skills, have a mental health problem, a substance abuse problem or a history of experiencing childhood abuse or neglect. Young et al. (2011, p. 899) state that, "parental emotional neglect is linked to psychiatric disorder". Bronfenbrenner's model is worth referring to, as described in more detail later in this chapter. Bronfenbrenner emphasises the existence of contexts in which parents interact with their children. Glaser (2011), on the other hand, emphasises that the caregiver-child relationship is embedded in a psychosocial context and that the clarity of understanding of the child's and the family's situation can be enhanced by analysing information according to the relevant tiers of concern.

Glaser points out the different contexts in which caregivers interact with children and how these contexts can contribute to emotional neglect. These contexts include family and environmental factors, as well as risk factors for caregivers such as mental health issues, substance abuse and childhood maltreatment. A study by Zhang et al. (2022, p. 9) showed

the relationship between childhood traumatic experiences and their intergenerational transmission; interestingly, they pointed out that our findings suggest that emotional neglect has a larger transmission effect than physical neglect, which makes the effects of different types of childhood trauma clearer.

Another model is the Environmental Deficit Model (Avdibegović & Brkić, 2020; Valtolina et al., 2023), which links this form of maltreatment to environmental and material deprivation. This model analyses how external phenomena such as poverty, social isolation, lack of community support or stressful living conditions contribute to neglect. Whereas, the ecological deficit model argues that these social and environmental phenomena can overwhelm parents, making it difficult for them to provide adequate care for their children. Also, the ecological-transactional model (Valtolina et al.,

2023) focuses on the continuous and reciprocal interaction between family characteristics and environment-related variables. It is the most holistic of the three models, integrating elements of the parental and environmental deficit models. It emphasises the dynamic interaction between parents, children and their wider environment. It recognises that both child and parent characteristics, as well as external phenomena and the quality of parent-child interactions, play a role in neglect.

Ecological systems theory (Bronfenbrenner, 1989) facilitates an understanding of the complexity of emotional neglect towards children in several ways and views the environment as an interactive set of systems that are "nested" within each other (Algood et al., 2011). Bronfenbrenner (1989) sees the environment as a system consisting of different interdependent levels: microsystem, mesosystem, exosystem and macrosystem. Each of these systems plays an important role in shaping the child's experience. The microsystem, or the child's immediate environment, includes direct interactions with parents, family members, school or peers. Here, the child experiences direct influences on his or her development. The mesosystem refers to the connections between the different microsystems, such as the home-school relationship. Although the exosystem does not involve direct interactions with the child, it influences the child through factors in which the child does not participate directly, such as the parent's workplace or local social policies. The macrosystem includes broad cultural, social, economic and political patterns influencing all other systems. *Therefore, child emotional neglect* is a complex phenomenon in which factors at every level of the ecological system play an important role. For example, parents' work-related stress (exosystem) can influence their behaviour towards children at home (microsystem). In turn, cultural norms and values (macrosystem) can shape family adherence to discipline and violence.

Family and socialisation of emotion

The main starting point in analysing the phenomenon of emotional neglect is the family environment, either natural or institutional, which plays an important role in the development of children and adolescents in shaping their life trajectories, although the institutional environment largely has a compensatory function). This has to do with the fact that a form of emotional neglect manifests itself primarily in the caregiver-child relationship, where, as already mentioned, the caregiver does not perceive or respect children's emotional needs appropriate to their age and developmental stage. The importance of the quality of relationships within the family, including the functioning of the family as a whole, satisfaction with family life and parent-child relationships, are key factors influencing the development of mental health problems in young adults (Saleem et al., 2021; Turner et al., 2006).

One of the family functions is emotional socialisation, presented in Eisenberg's heuristic model of the socialisation of emotion (2020, p. 655). Eisenberg's model provides an important tool in understanding the processes through which a child's emotions are shaped and transmitted in a social (including family) context. The model emphasises the importance of social and environmental interactions in children's emotional development, which is a key aspect of their overall development. According to this model, emotional modelling is one of the main mechanisms of emotional socialisation. Children learn to understand and express emotions by observing the behaviour of others, primarily parents and caregivers. For example, children often imitate the ways adults cope with stress or express joy. Therefore, parents have a key role in shaping their children's emotional patterns.

Another important aspect is the way adults react to the child's emotional expressions. These reactions can significantly impact how children will deal with their emotions in the future. For example, responding empathetically and supportively to a child's sadness can help develop healthy coping strategies to deal with negative emotions. Direct teaching and discussions about emotions are also an important part of the model. Parents and carers often teach children how to identify, understand and express emotions. Emotional education, including the teaching of the vocabulary of emotion, is considered crucial in helping children to understand better and communicate their feelings, which undoubtedly has an impact on their mental health. Positive socialisation of emotions can be a protective factor against emotional neglect and its negative consequences.

Although families differ in structure, parenting methods and behavioural models in different cultures, the institution of the family remains a key reference point in all human societies worldwide, especially in relation to the various phenomena within it (Bronfenbrenner, 1986). It is noteworthy that emotional neglect has intergenerational effects, affecting parental attitudes and the mental health of their children (Su et al., 2022). This model also highlights the role of transmitting cultural norms and values in socialising emotions. Different societies and cultures have different norms for expressing and experiencing emotions, which has an impact on a child's emotional development. Consequently, children raised in different cultural settings may develop different ways of understanding and expressing emotions (Eisenberg, 2020).

Not insignificant to emotional neglect, are the experiences of parents. Findings suggest that fathers' adverse childhood events may increase the risk of a child experiencing emotional neglect (Ylitervo et al., 2023). In contrast, research on the impact of childhood emotional neglect on motherhood shows that women who have experienced emotional neglect may have difficulty adapting to the changes associated with pregnancy and motherhood. This includes their relationship with their own bodies, as well as building a bond with their child and developing a sense of efficacy in their role as a mother.

Childhood emotional neglect can negatively impact a woman's ability to establish a positive relationship with her child (Talmon et al., 2019). Other studies have shown that emotional neglect by parents can result in several adverse effects, such as maladaptive coping mechanisms, a significant risk of becoming addicted to the internet (Salokangas et al., 2020; Sheng et al., 2022), elevated suicidal thoughts (Yu & Liu, 2020), limited self-discipline and deficient abilities in managing time effectively (Rees, 2008).

Social and cultural norms

The understanding of emotional neglect is influenced by the cultural context and social norms relating to parenting and the role of the carer. There are many different reasons why a parent may neglect his or her child, some of which can be very complex and result from a number of factors. One such factor is social norms influencing a person's individual thoughts and behaviour (Klika et al., 2019; Schultz et al., 2007). Social norms help determine what is correct and what is incorrect, what is typical or desirable. Two main types of norms are mentioned in the literature, descriptive norms are perceptions about what members of social groups do, while injunctive norms are perceptions about what members of a social group think others ought and ought not to do (Klika et al., 2019; Lilleston et al., 2017; Schultz et al., 2007).

It is worth noting that what is considered the norm in one society may not be acceptable in another. Such examples are cited by Lilleston et al. (2017, p. 124):

> In Peru, daughters have less economic potential compared to sons, which drives social norms permissive of parental neglect. In countries such as Sierra Leone and Guinea, with high prevalence of female genital mutilation, social norms related to the practice are strongly rooted in cultural and religious beliefs suggesting it enhances fertility and promotes female purity. Additionally, in South Asia, social norms related to child marriage are perpetuated by an entrenched system of patriarchy which denies women and girls rights to their own body and sexuality.

We can see common themes here, that is, cultural, economic and religious systems of norms affecting the lives and rights of children, in this case especially girls. Traditional beliefs can also be used to justify harmful practices, despite their negative impact on children's health and well-being. Witte and Mulla (2013, p. 960) note that:

> Individuals who misperceive the social norm by overestimating the prevalence of a particular behavior tend to engage in that behavior at an elevated frequency as if they were trying to bring their behavior in line with the norm.

An interesting example is given by Wessells and Kostelny (2021, p. 11), who point out that, "men in diverse contexts may expect that if they do not beat their wives, they will be criticised or ostracised by their male peers". Therefore, there is a link between social norms and emotional neglect. Wessells and Kostelny (2021) highlight the integral role of social norms in sustaining child neglect. Factors that make it challenging to learn about the phenomenon and fail to eliminate emotionally neglectful behaviour towards a child, effectively embody prevailing community norms and stereotypes regarding child-rearing, rules of obedience and the commonly prevailing "culture of violence". A culture of violence in the context of emotional neglect refers to an environment or value system in which the emotional needs of individuals are ignored or minimised. In such a culture, attention and resources may be focused on other aspects of life, such as material success or academic achievement, at the expense of emotional support, empathy and intimacy in interpersonal relationships.

Understanding the mechanisms by which these norms are perpetuated and altered is important for developing effective intervention and prevention strategies in the area of violence and neglect, as discussed more in Chapter 10.

Chapter 2

Invisibility in the spotlight

Pitfalls of understanding healthy development in the context of recent cultural changes

The right-thumb mentality

The contemporary world is facing a situation where the pace of socio-cultural changes outstrips the ability to adapt to new conditions. Many previously effective mechanisms supporting human development have lost their relevance. This is especially evident in the mental health field and necessitates a new perspective on models of health understanding.

The foundation of the considerations undertaken in this chapter is the mentality of the contemporary human being, based on five pillars: rationality, individualism, (high) technologisation, commercialism, and hedonism (Sikora & Górnik-Durose, 2013). This arrangement fosters a tendency towards behaviours like unambiguity, speed, and ease, which can be characterised as being similar to "swiping a thumb across a smartphone screen to make essential choices with a single tap". This mentality is referred to as the "right-thumb mentality".

Contemporary individuals are required to be rational, although the precise definition of rationality is often relegated to the background. This is tied to the other pillars of the right-thumb mentality. It suffices that our thinking or behaviour appears to be based on empirical evidence to be considered rational. The vast amount of knowledge we currently have access to makes it difficult to check everything that concerns us on our own. If something is labelled as "based on science" or "evidence-based", there is no perceived need to delve deeper; if advice appears to be evidence-based it can be followed. Conversely, being guided by irrationality (e.g., intuition or feeling) is deemed inappropriate and often dangerous. Reliance can only be placed on what is supported by a scientifically presenting authority.

Another pillar of the right-thumb mentality is individualism, which simultaneously forms the basis of democratic systems. In today's world, individuals are aware of their rights to self-determination, self-definition, and pursuing their own paths, often divergent from those shaped by their predecessors. Moving beyond inherited social forms and discovering one's own identity has become not just a value embedded in the ethos but virtually a

DOI: 10.4324/9781032621203-2

mandate (Giddens, 2006). This phenomenon leads to an urgent need to stand out among others and seek uniqueness, independence, and personal distinctiveness. Being ordinary is no longer satisfying. The desire to avoid these negative experiences drives searches, with the market responding by offering an ever-increasing array of personalised products. Personalisation is affecting more and more spheres of our lives. Not just insurance policies, diets, education or tailored medical treatments but personalised everyday items such as T-shirts, mugs, notebooks, or cars are increasingly desired (Sikora & Górnik-Durose, 2013). Technological progress, in turn, has opened up the possibility of limitless creation and self-expression in virtual space. Social networks and fandom[1] which bring the world of fantasy into reality basically allow for free expression and the transcending of physical limitations, so that you can be whoever you want. The main issue may be one of standing out among billions of other internet users. Previously, social comparisons involved a relatively small group of people – peers, members of the local community, acquaintances from school, work, or vacations, so it was easier to differentiate oneself. Now, social comparisons involve not only a significantly increased number of people but also "unfair" competition due to the impossibility of verifying the information posted by users online.

Access to new technologies, infinite Internet resources, and networks of contacts on social media mean that the need to differentiate or craft oneself and one's opinion may grow even further. New ideas and new areas to explore come along with increasingly more information that must be assimilated and kept up with. On the one hand, fast and broad access to information can make life easier and often help solve complex issues; on the other hand, it can lead to tension and anxiety, fearing we might overlook something crucial and fall out of the loop. FOMO (fear of missing out) is spreading more widely among people in the 21st century. A rational person cannot easily dismiss something so useful. Technological progress means that information circulates incredibly quickly. The evolution of mobile phones, and now smartphones, shows that these solutions have not only enabled easy contact between people from almost all over the world but have also introduced new communication rules. Delays in responding to calls or messages become unforgivable, and the possibility of contact anytime and anywhere means that the expectation of autonomy is reduced. In contrast, the area of control is expanded. The ability to share information instantly, which becomes outdated amidst a flood of other information within a few hours or even minutes, increases the risk of exclusion. It is easy to shift interpersonal activity from reality to the virtual world. Meanwhile, the overload of information to process reduces the chance for in-depth analysis. Drawing conclusions, thinking abstractly, and processing data at a meta-level becomes more challenging. As Bauman (2009) writes, situations begin to be perceived as a collection of issues lacking depth or essence (see Sikora & Górnik-Durose, 2013).

Technological progress also facilitates the development of the retail sector. New devices and equipment require new behaviours, often leading to the purchase of new resources – protective covers for devices, clothing, gadgets, cloud storage, etc. Limited support for specific models of hardware or software forces their replacement after some time, even though an individual may not feel the need for such change. Existing behavioural patterns are also evolving. Global Positioning System (GPS) eliminates the need to ask for directions, and shopping through apps allows for contactless transactions. More and more areas of human life, including its most private zones, are becoming commercialised. Brands become indicators of sought-after values and satisfied needs, making people create their identities by acquiring them. Possessing certain goods is supposed to ensure happiness, relationship success and self-confidence. Commercialised customs, such as the obligation to give gifts to loved ones on occasions not only of major events but also on holidays created specifically for this purpose, like Valentine's Day, Cat Day, Kiss A Ginger Day, or Hamburger Day, mean that lack of engagement on these days can be treated as a sign of lack of affection, social indifference or withdrawal. Finally, the ability to buy experiences fits into the phenomenon of affluenza (de Graaf et al., 2005), the contagion of prosperity among people, the desire to possess an ever-increasing amount of goods to match others, and to achieve success on the scale of the "American dream". Meanwhile, the well-documented hedonic treadmill in positive psychology (see Diener et al., 2006) means that we get used to accumulating goods and experiences; they no longer bring joy, and we again need something more.

Deriving pleasure from life has never been as accessible as it is now. The pursuit of pleasure and discomfort seems natural to humans. However, in the 21st century, this pursuit has become universally obligatory and increasingly justified culturally. Happiness has become the most important goal, with technological and consumer possibilities allowing discomfort avoidance. There is a trend towards making daily activities easier and more enjoyable, including work, transport, education, healthcare, cleaning or doing the dishes. Contemporary hedonism, however, requires rationalisation; it is measurable, profitable, fast and easy, demanding pleasure to be drawn from the right sources and in the correct way, grounded in expert knowledge, promoted and approved in the social groups we live in (Giddens, 2006).

Contemporary (non)understanding of health

Considering the pillars of right-thumb mentality, let us look at the issue of contemporary understanding of health. We live in an era of maximisation – surrounded by an all-encompassing desire to achieve the greatest benefits in the shortest possible time: material, emotional, experiential and also health-related. We want to be healthier and live as long as possible with the highest quality of life. However, defining health, including mental health, has become an enormous challenge today. Health is a value in itself, as well as an instrumental value, being a condition for a satisfying life, happiness, development, social acceptance, attractiveness, etc. The most firmly established models of health understanding in the empirical context – biomedical and biopsychosocial – have long since ceased to fulfil their explanatory and predictive functions (Wojtyna & Stawiarska, 2013). It is time to critically examine them and introduce new perspectives enriched with aspects relevant to contemporary humans.

Contemporary obstacles to the biomedical model of health

The biomedical model of health defines *health* as the absence of disease (Sheridan & Radmacher, 1998), focusing not so much on health itself but rather on disease and disorder. In somatic medicine, it is relatively easy to determine what is dysfunctional and life-threatening to the organism's functioning. The goal of medical interventions here is the correction of abnormalities or deviations. A *disease state* can be defined as the presence of symptoms or other visible or detectable signs of organ and system function impairment. An expert in this field, typically a doctor with the appropriate knowledge and qualifications, is deemed competent to assess these symptoms. However, difficulties arise when applying such an approach to mental health. The long-standing issue of diagnosing health or mental disorders is based on the use of norm definitions, including quantitative, socio-cultural, and theoretical norms. However, none of these norms clearly distinguishes between a state of health and disease and 21st-century individual struggles with ambiguity. This translates into an intense search for increasingly sophisticated "normality" criteria, with a growing number of experts, not just doctors, participating in their determination. The media undoubtedly plays a role as an accelerator and catalyst for these trends (Roy, 2008).

The result of these phenomena is medicalisation, or the defining of natural, physiological processes in pathological terms, which leads to the search for therapeutic methods to correct the problem (Conrad, 2007). This is particularly evident in the context of mood disorders, where feelings of unhappiness, transient mood dips, or grief may be perceived as a health problem and associated with depression, requiring pharmacological or psychotherapeutic support, especially since current versions of classification systems for mental illnesses and disorders (DSM-5 – Diagnostic and Statistical Manual of Mental Disorders, 5th Edition and CD-11- International Classification of Diseases, 11th Revision) allow for the diagnosis of a depressive episode after just two weeks of persistent symptoms. Difficulties with attention may be associated with Attention Deficit Hyperactivity Disorder (ADHD), irritability and impulsivity with borderline personality disorders, and lessened mental flexibility with neuroatypicality within the autism spectrum. This trend towards medicalisation can be fuelled by the desire for commercial success by drug or supplement manufacturers who seek to attract ever-wider swathes of customers and, under the guise of rationality – a pillar of contemporary mentality – encourage the diagnosis of a problem and the use of a tailored treatment programme. Undoubtedly, a positive effect of medicalisation is the creation of an opportunity for individuals to justify their problems in medical terms, which allows them to protect their self-image and attempt to free themselves from perceived discomfort (Cacchioni & Wolkowitz, 2011). In line with the "can do" culture, since the tools exist, it would be irrational not to take advantage of their benefits (Paris, 2015). However, rationality requires a "serious" approach to the issue, so we need a diagnosis. This need, along with the fear of patient litigiousness and the fear of overlooking significant health problems, prompts doctors towards overdiagnosis. Making a false-positive diagnosis is better than missing a severe illness (Paris, 2015). Thus, the widespread use of methylphenidate or amphetamine by individuals with attention difficulties under the guise of ADHD (Franco et al., 2020) is not surprising. We reach for antidepressants to rid ourselves of a bad mood and for drugs like modafinil to mitigate fatigue. There is a medicine for every symptom, and for every medicine a new indication can be found (Busfield, 2010; Triggle, 2007).

Meanwhile, advances in diagnostics enable the identification of existing dysfunctions and pathologies before their symptoms appear clinically. This raises questions: Is implementing treatment at such an early, preclinical stage sensible? Does the balance of potential benefits outweigh the treatment's adverse actions and side effects? The difficulty of tolerating uncertainty favours the implementation of treatment to avoid potential future patient claims.

Challenges for a biopsychosocial approach to health

Despite the difficulties mentioned above, the biomedical model of health can still defend its position in somatic health. However, it is much more challenging to find objective indicators of the absence of disease in relation to mental health. Here, the biopsychosocial approach offers more assistance. According to the *World Health Organization* (WHO), *health* in this context is defined as a "state of complete physical, mental and social well-being and not merely the absence of disease or infirmity" (World Health Organization). Meanwhile, in Antonovsky's (1979) salutogenic approach, health is understood in procedural terms – the search for and maintenance of balance in the face of stressors encountered by the human organism. Disease here signifies the failure of this process. Finally, the definition of health derived from the health promotion field describes it as "a person's evolving ability to achieve their full physical, psychological, and social potential and to respond to environmental challenges" (Słońska & Misiuna, 1993, p. 68).

The biopsychosocial, holistic approach to health seemingly appears more adequate and possesses more significant predictive and explanatory power than the biomedical model. However, this is misleading (Wojtyna & Stawiarska, 2013). How can well-being be operationalised? Where does balance lie, and when is it achieved? Moreover, where is the elusive peak of our capabilities? Contemporary socio-cultural changes and technological advancements also confuse the categories of holistic health understanding. There is no clear unambiguous definition of health behaviours. What benefits one person may harm another, and the line between pro- and anti-health behaviours becomes incredibly thin.

One of the most frequently cited examples of health behaviour that can become both a health-supporting and damaging activity is engaging in physical activity. There is undeniable evidence of the positive impact of physical activity on somatic and mental health. However, on the flip side, excessive involvement in training can lead to injuries, damage, and even addiction (Caponnetto et al., 2021; Weinstein & Szabo, 2023). For example, physical exercises are part of the clinical expression of eating disorders (Rizk et al., 2020). Moreover, the increased incidence of anorexia, bulimia or bigorexia is associated with excessive care for the body and its appearance (see Mosley, 2009; Neumark-Sztainer et al., 2006; Vasiliu, 2023). These disorders often coincide with pharmacological agents and medical procedures that may support achieving the ideal body image (Pope et al., 2005). Meanwhile, an excessive focus on healthy eating (intensively promoted by media and marketing) often turns into orthorexia (Mahfoud et al., 2023; Valente et al., 2022).

Taking care of one's health is ingrained in the rational and empirical thinking of the responsible 21st-century individual. Here again, the significant role of the media is evident. Through numerous strategies, often messages that induce fear, the media directs us to take responsibility for our health and the health of our loved ones (see Polzer & Knabe, 2012; Roy, 2008). The attempt to reduce anxiety and uncertainty makes us more willing to engage in behaviours proposed and promoted as rational. However, we don't always know what is truly rational, and the risk of making the wrong decision paralyses us. This is part of the phenomenon of decision regret and anticipatory regret or fear of better options (FOBO) or fear of doing anything (FODA) (Gigerenzer & Garcia-Retamero, 2017; Schwartz & Ward, 2004). Is the decision to (or not) get vaccinated against COVID-19 the right one? – this question recently confronted humanity in the face of the SARS-CoV-2 pandemic. The modern world expects us to make responsible decisions. However, the amount of information and data that need to be analysed is almost infinite. It is no wonder then that people fall into the trap of counterfactual thinking. It is becoming increasingly difficult for contemporary individuals to take responsibility for their health and its treatment, while it is becoming easier to immerse in what Seligman called learned helplessness (Seligman, 1974). Thus, existing models of understanding health are becoming more and more outdated.

"Right-thumb" approach to health – the ideal correction and total development

The 21st-century human, thanks to advancements in science and technology, is capable of developing in virtually any direction and transcending boundaries that were once set by biological or material factors. This opens up possibilities that allow shifting the norm indicator on the illness-health continuum. Consequently, health begins to be perceived not only as a "possibility", but as a state of "maintaining" the peak of one's physical, psychological, and social capabilities (Wojtyna & Stawiarska, 2013). In addition, the spiritual dimension is increasingly included in holistic health definitions. However, this trend has a more quantitative than qualitative dimension, which aligns with the maximisation drive embedded in contemporary human mentality. This leads to an intensification of the "pathology versus ideal health" dichotomy, causing behaviours undertaken in the area of health to focus on the one hand on correcting every sign of defect or pathology, even those insignificant from a medical standpoint, and on the other hand on striving to reach the peak of one's capabilities, that is total self-development. Medicine becomes not only therapy but also a vehicle for self-improvement (Clark et al., 2003; Coveney et al., 2011). Correcting crooked teeth becomes the norm even when the perceived irregularities are not considered bite defects. Increasingly, aesthetic and plastic surgery procedures are undertaken in children. There are also tendencies to prosthesis, repair, and rehabilitate every physical defect, which may allow children to develop physically better, but often at the expense of development in other life areas.

Pursuing an ideal quality of life and perfect health also involves comprehensive physical, psychological, social, and spiritual development. However, the "right-thumb" mentality pushes us towards quick and unambiguous solutions, which are often in conflict with the traditional understanding of development. This makes living at 100% in a given area of functioning the only measure that unequivocally indicates a job well done.

Efforts to expand health resources are supported by the contemporary actions of sports organisations, scientific bodies, local communities and non-governmental organisations (e.g., open sports events), as well as phenomena observed on social media and online platforms. Many influencers and online communities organise open channels and events that promote health-oriented behaviours. These activities can support the motivation to adopt and maintain healthy habits (Carr et al., 2013; Davies et al., 2012); however, there are several pitfalls. One of these is the challenges posted online, which may lead to engaging in activities that are inadvisable for health reasons or may lead to excessive activity. Meanwhile, competition may foster a desire to earn another trophy (even if only in the form of likes, a place in the rankings, or a virtual badge), rather than genuine health considerations. This acquisition of new experiences mirrors the affluenza phenomenon observed in consumer behaviours (De Graaf et al., 2005). Accumulated trophies, completed marathons, and attended spiritual development workshops become new status indicators for social groups. Meanwhile, the need to assert one's individuality supports actions that enhance the possibility of being noticed and recognised. The increasing technicisation of health activities, requiring the acquisition of specialised equipment, appropriate footwear for a given sport, and the healthiest food products, exacerbates social inequalities due to economic status differences (James, 2007). Health has become a domain for wealthy people. Even if someone breaks away from affluenza-driven trends, they often need to clearly define their behaviour, thus creating a new or reinforcing another trend (e.g., slow food, slow jogging, and minimalism). Health behaviours are increasingly entering a space previously reserved for self-presentation (Karelas, 2011).

Today, pushing our limits is not just about increasing our physical, intellectual, spiritual, or emotional capacity. A transhumanist path has opened before us, leading beyond the boundaries set by nature (Bostrom, 2005). It is worth noting that, according to the concept of the "brain-artefact interface" (BAI), sensory extensions through technology lead to neuroplastic changes in the brain, consequently altering perception, ways of thinking, and human functioning in the world (Malafouris, 2010). However, even the decision to utilise the opportunities provided by science and technology or to accept natural limitations is not straightforward. Transcending natural boundaries, as well as remaining within them, are mutually exclusive, while the benefits and risks are precisely reversed in each of these options.

Nevertheless, accepting natural limitations remains in conflict with the right-thumb rule of maximisation and unambiguity. It seems more rational to strive to exploit contemporary scientific achievements, pharmacotherapy and technology to increase one's chances, as this allows for achieving a greater number (maximisation) of comparable (unambiguous) results and objectives (Gazzaniga, 2008; Hughes, 2004; Wojtyna & Stawiarska, 2013).

In physicality, this would mean developing one's endurance, physical fitness, and shaping the body through both natural capabilities and the aid of technological achievements or various substances. This also fits into the quick and straightforward solutions that are expectations of the right-thumb mentality. It is noticeable that climbing the world's highest peaks, overcoming challenging distances, or functioning in extremely harsh weather conditions is no longer a problem. Thanks to technology, we can do what has resulted in the deaths of daredevils until recently. There is also an increase in the use of substances that support the development of physique, muscle mass, and nutritional substances to improve body appearance. The popularity of aesthetic medicine and plastic surgery procedures is also rising. However, it is essential to consider the identity aspect of body modifications. Such modifications, including tattoos, piercings, scarification, and even amputations or insertion of implants, can serve functions that symbolically emphasise the seriousness of certain events or someone's individuality or, conversely, belonging to a significant social group for the individual (Carmen et al., 2012).

There are many opportunities for improvement in mental functioning, such as effective methods for training cognitive functions and developing creativity, memory and concentration. We have developed effective psychotherapeutic methods that allow for better emotion regulation and mood improvement. However, these methods are neither easy nor quick, which contradicts the right-thumb mentality. Solutions that offer rapid results may be more attractive. These include increasingly accessible artificial intelligence tools, Internet resources, and psychoactive and pharmacological substances.

The use of coffee and energy drinks in situations of fatigue has already become the norm. There has also been increased social awareness regarding the medically safe use of psychostimulants to improve attention concentration in diagnosed cases of ADHD in adults. Available meta-analyses indicate that single doses of psychostimulants improve cognitive functioning in healthy individuals (Becker et al., 2022). However, the use of psychostimulants to enhance mental abilities beyond norms remains controversial. Similar dilemmas involve the use of substances such as psilocybin or oxytocin to improve spiritual or social functioning. There is plenty of empirical evidence that externally administered oxytocin can enhance prosocial behaviours and strengthen empathy, trust, or willingness to sacrifice for others (Zak et al., 2005). Meanwhile, psilocybin is an example of a psychoactive substance that allows for mystical experiences, but also supports a long-term altruistic and prosocial attitude (Griffiths et al., 2011). However, a problem arises: does enhancing human mental abilities through the use of psychoactive substances truly fit into right-thumb maximisation and individualism? Perhaps the complications that may emerge as a result of such actions will become pathologies, fitting into the biomedical model of health understanding and requiring further correction. People risk falling into a vicious cycle where improvement in one area necessitates the continual correction of emerging complications.

Summarising the considerations so far, in both fundamental models of understanding health – biomedical and biopsychosocial – there are tendencies to develop increasingly sensitive indicators of health and illness, as well as tendencies to support health with more sophisticated methods. As a result, it becomes possible to expand health, but this happens at the potential expense of mutually cannibalising actions. It is impossible to correct everything, just as it is impossible to develop in all areas of life. We are limited by natural factors (such as time and ageing), environmental factors (such as disasters like the COVID-19 pandemic), or economic factors (because we cannot afford everything available). These limitations lead to frustration and chronic stress, which worsens the broadly understood quality of life. The mounting distress and chronicity of this process can, in turn, trigger further disturbing symptoms considered pathological and requiring further correction. We are liable to fall into the trap of a vicious circle, as illustrated in Figure 2.1.

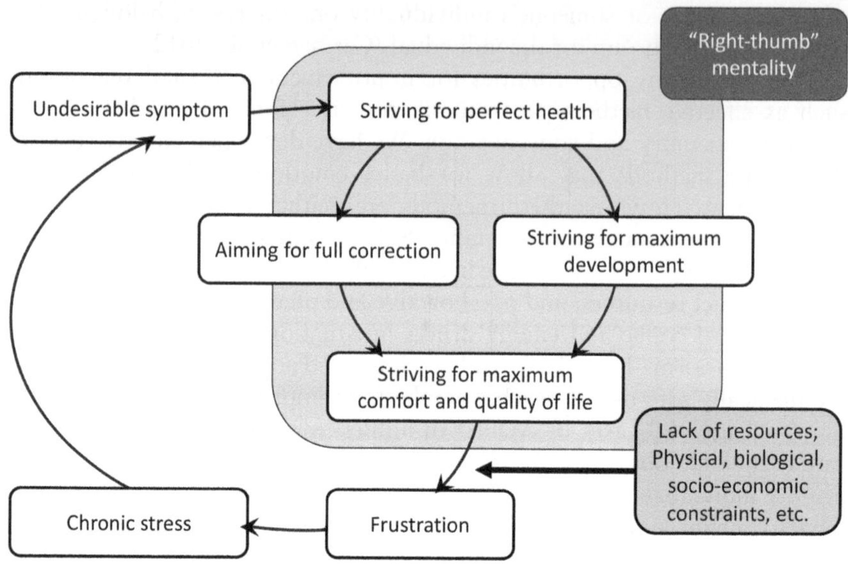

Figure 2.1 The vicious circle of the "right-thumb" understanding of health.

The above-mentioned vicious cycle in the right-thumb mentality's understanding of health will become the canvas for further considerations undertaken in this book. This vicious circle consumes time, material and energy resources and can lead to serious emotional neglect in close relationships, because it is impossible to implement the ideal assumptions that the right-thumb mentality imposes on a person, including (or perhaps especially) a parent in the 21st century.

Note

1 Fandom is a term that refers to a community of fans who share a common interest in a particular subject, such as a literary work, film, TV series, video game, sport or artist. These communities engage in various activities, such as discussions, creating fan art, writing fan fiction, organising meetups, and participating in conventions. Fandoms often develop their own subcultures and traditions, fostering a sense of belonging and shared identity among their members.

Chapter 3

The social brain

Neurobiological and evolutionary mechanisms related to neglect

The "right thumb mentality" described in the previous chapter focuses attention on the individual. However, humans are inherently social creatures, evolutionarily derived from herd animals and still living within a network of social contacts. Numerous studies have shown that a satisfying social life is a predictor of both physical and mental health (Pearce et al., 2017; Schmälzle et al., 2017). Consequently, the ability to adapt to complex mechanisms at the interface between the individual and the social system becomes a significant challenge for anyone who wants to survive and maintain a good quality of life.

Social brain theory

Humans, as a species, achieve independence quite late since children are completely dependent on adult care for many years (Brüne, 2016). This dependency requires the intense involvement of parents or caregivers in processes that meet the child's needs and provide the resources necessary for development. Among the many needs that must be satisfied, this book focuses on a few that are particularly important for human development and well-being, namely the need for safety, autonomy, competence, self-worth and relationships with others (Ryan & Deci, 2017). Young et al. (2003) highlighted another crucial emotional need for children, which is essential for forming healthy functional social patterns – having established boundaries. Some of these needs, such as the need for autonomy and relationships with others, may seem contradictory or, as Roediger et al. (2018) wrote, represent two poles of one dimension. Therefore, an important developmental task is to find a flexible balance between these needs. Failure to satisfy these needs signifies a state of threat to the organism, leading to stress and initiation of compensatory reactions (Cannon, 2016). These reactions include fights (undertaken when there is a chance to gain autonomy, control, or dominance), flights (aimed at actively avoiding danger and achieving relief), freeze responses (withdrawing from a threatening situation through emotional detachment, dissociation and/or numbness), and fawning (where one follows or submits to an adversary in

DOI: 10.4324/9781032621203-3

order to remain part of a group or maintain a bond). Meanwhile, the search for a balance between autonomy and living in a larger social group mirrors the situation that our ancestors had to navigate through evolution.

The survival and reproduction mechanisms developed in ancient times for hominins and so-called anatomically modern humans are still relevant to the brain of the 21st-century human. Thus, despite the advancements in civilisation and sociocultural changes, many of our social behaviours are governed by the same principles that our ancestors developed. This is related to what is known as evolutionary lag, which involves genetic changes occurring at a pace that is incomparably slower than changes in the environment where the selection process takes place (Buss, 2015). Evolution favoured individuals who were capable of forming strong social bonds. By building well-functioning social networks, our ancient ancestors increased their chances of survival and reproduction. The processing of phenomena occurring in relationships with others must therefore be reflected in changes in brain structure.

Forming larger social groups increased hominins' chances of defending against predators, but also heightened competition for food and sexual partners, necessitating further ventures in search of sustenance. The cost of greater safety was the increased stress associated with new challenges in relationships among social group members. Evolutionary psychology posits that most human brain functions are not related to solving abstract problems, but rather focus on social problems (Cosmides, 1989). The Social Brain Theory (Brothers, 2002) links the increase in hominins' brain size, especially in the frontal lobes, with the expansion of social networks to sizes where individuals could minimise the conflict between autonomy and group life. While the optimal group size for apes is approximately several dozen individuals, for humans it has been estimated to be approximately 150 people, known as Dunbar's number (Dunbar & Schultz, 2007; Lindenfors et al., 2021). However, it seems that the actual size of a group is less important than the social complexity, which manifests as the ability to form complex relationships based on mutual cooperation (Dunbar & Schultz, 2007). In turn, this requires the development of an excellent empathic understanding of both one's own and others' mental and emotional states. Empathy is a complex concept and can thus be defined in various ways. For the purpose of this book, we focus on two aspects of understanding the mental states of others: affective and cognitive.

The affective dimension of empathy involves the capacity to intuitively respond to other people's emotions (Zaki & Ochsner, 2012). This often includes the phenomenon of emotional contagion, where one automatically responds to the emotions of others with the same reaction without understanding the contextual factors that elicit the original emotion (Gonzalez-Liencres et al., 2013). Through empathy, one can evoke both basic emotions, such as joy, sadness, fear, surprise, and disgust/contempt, as well as complex emotions, such as shame, guilt, envy and schadenfreude (i.e. pleasure derived from another's misfortune or failure). However, it is necessary to decode social signals transmitted through facial expressions, gestures and body posture. This dimension of empathy can also be found in animals.

On the other hand, the cognitive dimension of empathy, which is specific to humans, can be linked to mentalisation, otherwise known as theory of mind. This is the ability to reflect on the mental states of oneself and others in terms of intentions, needs, beliefs, etc. The ability to mentalise develops in the early years of life, but it is only around the age of 3 to 4 years that a child acquires the ability to distinguish their own beliefs about the world from those of another person, while by the age of 5 to 6 years, the child begins to understand that someone can have beliefs about another person's beliefs. The development of the theory of mind is closely related to the bond between the child and parent (Hughes & Ensor, 2006; von Klitzing et al., 1999) and progresses more smoothly and quickly when caregivers frequently use terms describing their own and others mental and emotional states during conversations with the child. The presence of older siblings, peers, and other children can also accelerate the development of mentalisation. It is also important to remember that culture can modulate the timing and speed of social competency development (Greenfield et al., 2003). The developmental processes related to these issues will be discussed more broadly in subsequent chapters of the book.

The neural basis of empathy and mentalisation

The development of empathic and mentalisation competencies is associated with the development of specific areas of the central nervous system. Neuronal networks that process emotions are primarily linked to the medial cortex of the cingulate gyrus and limbic areas such as the amygdala and insula (Lamm et al., 2007). The crucial role of the amygdala in building and maintaining social networks through the processing of nonverbal stimuli that occur during interactions with other people, such as gestures or facial expressions, has been repeatedly demonstrated (Bickart et al., 2012; Jones et al., 2020). A larger volume and greater density of grey matter in the amygdala not only enhance the reading of complex social signals, but also make interactions with others seem more attractive, thereby easing the maintenance and formation of new social relationships (Bickart et al., 2012; Liu et al., 2019; Zerubavel et al., 2015).

The amygdala performs its functions in conjunction with other brain areas. Functional connections with the orbitofrontal cortex (OFC) enable face recognition, social reward processing, and engagement in prosocial behaviours (Hampton et al., 2016; Kwak et al., 2018). Interestingly, the connection between the amygdala and the OFC facilitates the analysis of scent, a social signal that carries information about another person, such as foreignness, threats, or possible diseases. For instance, it is known that mothers and children can recognise each other through scent, and even unrelated individuals such as romantic partners or friends can do so (Leschak & Eisenberger, 2018). This may explain the tendency to isolate individuals who emit an unpleasant odour. It is not merely an aesthetic issue, but may stem from evolutionarily developed adaptive processes related to avoiding contact with potentially threatening individuals, such as those who are toxic, infected, or sick. Greater olfactory sensitivity, linked with the connection between the amygdala and the OFC, translates into a larger social network size constructed by the individual (Zou et al., 2016).

Meanwhile, functions encompassed by the theory of mind are associated with activation of what is called the mentalisation network, which consists of neuronal circuits, including the medial prefrontal cortex (mPFC), medial orbitofrontal cortex (mOFC), posterior cingulate cortex (pCC), precuneus, right temporoparietal junction (TPJ), and areas containing mirror neurons (Behrens et al., 2008; Frith & Frith, 2001; Hanakawa et al., 2003; Mitchell, 2009; Molenberghs et al., 2016; Morishima et al., 2012; Muscatell et al., 2012; Tusche et al., 2016). The ventromedial prefrontal cortex (vmPFC) and OFC are responsible for understanding the emotional states of others, whereas the dorsomedial PFC (dmPFC) and dorsolateral PFC (dlPFC) are involved in inferring the intentions and beliefs of others (Abu-Akel & Shamay-Tsoory, 2011; Han et al., 2021). The function of the right temporoparietal junction (rTPJ) is linked to understanding the false mental states of others and reorienting attention; that is, the ability to shift attention to unexpected stimuli. Mirror neurons represent an important neuronal system that aids in mimicking and understanding the actions of others (Ikeda et al., 2019). This system includes the inferior frontal gyrus (IFG), inferior parietal lobule (IPL), and the posterior superior temporal sulcus (pSTS). The latter area is particularly crucial for analysing and mimicking social signals, such as eye, mouth and body movements (Deen & Saxe, 2019). There is a proportional relationship between the activation of the pSTS and the size of social networks formed (Dziura & Thompson, 2014; Han et al., 2021; Kirby et al., 2018).

Close relationships in the "right-thumb" social brain

The right-thumb mentality's quest for uniqueness and drive to maximise effects are closely linked to enhancing social status. Studies have shown that social status is associated on the one hand with the development of neuronal networks that process information about interpersonal interactions, while on the other hand, it is connected to the structure of social networks. Individuals with lower socioeconomic status show lower grey matter density in the frontal, temporal, and parietal cortices, hippocampus, and amygdala (Brito & Noble, 2014; Willard & Shively, 2016). A higher social status facilitates the development of social networks. However, it is important to note that in the modern world, individuals with high social status tend to have a larger number of social relationships, but their involvement in close relationships can be significantly reduced or limited to very few contacts. Meanwhile, individuals with lower socioeconomic status may have fewer social relations, but these may be of higher quality (Han et al., 2021). Recall that the human brain, according to Dunbar's number, may struggle to process more than 150 close relationships.

We can further develop the right-thumb model of health using the phenomena described above (Figure 3.1). The pursuit of as many high-quality relationships as possible is associated with the overload of neuronal networks related to empathy and mentalisation. In turn, this can lead to a decrease in

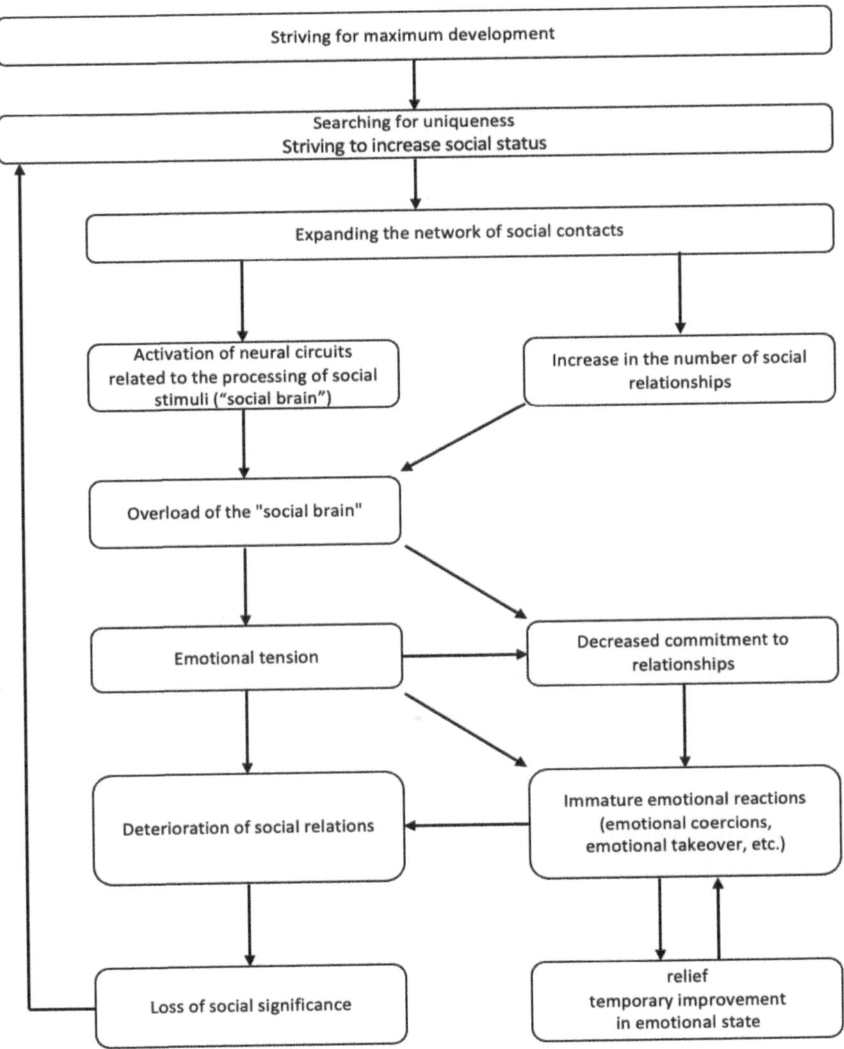

Figure 3.1 Right-thumb striving for development and the social brain.

engagement in relationships and an increase in emotional tension, which the individual will try to discharge. The attempt to discharge and simultaneously maintain many relationships can lead to the activation of immature emotional reactions such as emotional coercion or emotional takeover (Gibson, 2019). Discharge leads to temporary relief, which may reinforce these emotional reactions. However, in the long term, this leads to the deterioration of social relationships and loss of status, which, in turn, intensifies compensatory attempts to prove one's uniqueness and high status.

The chemistry of close relationships

The ability to create and maintain close bonds is also regulated by substances, such as oxytocin, dopamine, and beta-endorphins (Pearce et al., 2017). Oxytocin, a neuropeptide, participates in the formation of bonds between partners as well as in the parent-child relationship and regulates the transmission of socio-emotional information, including emotional contagion among people (Insel et al., 2001; Spengler et al., 2017; Yoshida et al., 2009). Oxytocin promotes sensitivity to socially relevant signals. Its effect on the autonomic nervous system facilitates inhibition of the stress response at the level of the hypothalamus-pituitary-adrenal axis. Interestingly, by stimulating the C-tactile fibres present in the hairy skin, oxytocin secretion occurs as a result of affiliative touch interactions. The "social touch" hypothesis suggests that this is a mechanism analogous to grooming observed in animals, which strengthens social bonds between individuals in a group (Dunbar, 2010; Handlin et al., 2023; Morrison et al., 2010). Touch, which activates C-tactile fibres, signals the proximity of other important people and fosters a sense of security. The most effective stress-relieving social touch occurs with movements at speeds ranging from 1 to 10 cm/s (Ackerley et al., 2014; Löken et al., 2009). Repeated studies have shown that intranasal administration of oxytocin strengthens social relations, encourages affiliative behaviours, enhances trust, and intensifies emotional transmission (Spengler et al., 2017; Xu et al., 2019;).

Dopamine is a neurotransmitter present in circuits related to theory of mind (Abu-Akel & Shamay-Tsoory, 2011) and affects many areas of the brain, including the amygdala, ventromedial prefrontal cortex, and anterior cingulate cortex (Atzil et al., 2017), which are areas associated with empathy. Disorders in dopaminergic circuits, such as in schizophrenia and autism, are linked to a reduced capacity for empathic responses in social interactions. Atzil et al. (2017) showed that maternal bonding and a sense of social belonging depend on dopaminergic reward circuits. Previously mentioned social touch, which fosters oxytocin release, has been found in recent studies to potentially stimulate dopamine secretion in the mesolimbic reward system through gentle social touch (Elias & Abdus-Saboor, 2022; Elias et al., 2023).

Finally, the endorphin system is essential for maintaining stable social relationships and for experiencing attachment and social warmth (Machin & Dunbar, 2011; Pearce et al., 2017). The relationship between the opioid system and social connections is bidirectional. Beta-endorphins participate in perceiving the positive value of social relationships and promoting a larger social network built by an individual (Johnson & Dunbar, 2016). In turn, close relationships encourage the release of endorphins. Interestingly, if the activities that promote endorphin release are performed together, the effects of endogenous opioids are enhanced. In primates, activation of the endorphin system is triggered by social grooming (Keverne et al., 1989); however, similar mechanisms have also been demonstrated in the human brain, especially in the frontal lobe (Dunbar, 2022; Nummenmaa et al., 2018). Additionally, activities performed together to strengthen endorphin release include laughter and collective music-making, singing, or dancing as well as rituals performed in a group, such as religious rituals or those associated with significant events in a particular social group. Laughter is considered a vocal analogue of grooming, but it is faster and can involve a larger group of people, significantly speeding up and facilitating the building of social bonds. Finally, endorphins participate in the reduction of both physical and social pain.

Pain of a broken heart

Social pain is the phenomenon of experiencing physical pain in response to social stimuli associated with abandonment, exclusion, unfair treatment, or loss of a close relationship (Eisenberger et al., 2006). In many languages around the world, such experiences are described using terms that denote physical injury, such as "broken heart" or "hurt feelings" (MacDonald & Leary, 2005). This is due to the overlap of neuronal circuits responsible for processing social relationship information with those responsible for nociception (Eisenberger & Lieberman, 2004; Eisenberger et al., 2003). From an evolutionary perspective, pain is one of the strongest alarm signals, and disconnection from the herd is a situation threatening an individual's survival. In this context, the overlay of networks processing "exclusion from the herd" signals and those related to the conduction of physical pain information (including dACC, anterior insula, periaqueductal grey, nucleus accumbens, striatum) makes profound sense (Chester et al., 2012). Eisenberger et al. (2003) demonstrated that individuals experiencing a laboratory-induced sense of rejection (through the Cyberball game, in which the participant is ignored in a virtual ball-tossing game) show activation of neuronal circuits associated with nociception and an increased sensitivity to pain. It has also been shown that in the face of threat, pain thresholds and tolerance decrease (Bernstein & Claypool, 2012; DeWall & Baumeister, 2006; Wojtyna et al., 2024). Interestingly, individuals who experience chronic social rejection and are characterised by fragile self-esteem (high explicit and low implicit self-esteem) may, in situations of acute social threat, exhibit an increased pain threshold while also showing an intensified stress response (Wojtyna et al., 2024). Similarly, DeWall and Baumeister (2006) found that social exclusion can reduce sensitivity to physical pain. However, this seemingly contradictory phenomenon to the concept of social pain can be explained by adaptive transient analgesia, which is induced by high-intensity stimuli (Alter et al., 2020; Gear et al., 1999; Grill & Coghill, 2002).

The phenomenon of social pain may be significantly Intensified in current times. The dominance of individualism, competitiveness, or the need to achieve as many goals as possible in the shortest time promotes behaviours that deviate from fair play. Relational losses, which activate social pain circuits, may also be associated with the phenomenon of social isolation resulting from the virtualisation of interpersonal contacts. This is influenced not only by the increasingly remote mode of work arrangements but also by remote forms of education. The transfer of social relationships to an online version expanded during the COVID-19 pandemic and is still being continued owing to increasingly developing technologies. Jauch et al. (2022) showed that even in a human-computer relationship, social exclusion by a non-human factor leads to increasing social pain.

Given that social phenomena, associated with social neglect and behaviours far from fair play influence the sensation of pain and activation of the endorphin system in the central nervous system, it should not be surprising that there is an abuse of painkillers, including opioids. The opioid epidemic is claiming an increasing number of lives worldwide. Fentanyl is known to kill younger people and physically healthy individuals (Gaur et al., 2020; Lyons et al., 2019; Wilson et al., 2020). It is possible that opioid abuse is indeed due to social pain and growing difficulties in social relationships. Activation of the endorphin system allows not only achieving an analgesic effect but also eliminating the affective component of pain and the maintaining of a large network of social contacts. However, the costs of these benefits can be fatally serious.

Neglect in close relationships, associated with a threat to health and life, leads to chronic stress and mental and somatic health problems, including social pain, depressive disorders, and other neuropsychiatric issues (Eisenberger, 2012; Giotakos, 2020; Reilly & Gunnar, 2019). In subsequent chapters, we will take a closer look at emotional neglect and its consequences on well-being and mental health at various developmental stages of children and adolescents.

Emotional neglect and 21st-century human: continuity of evolutionary and biological mechanisms

Despite cultural and technological advancements, humans in the 21st century remain under the strong influence of evolutionary and biological mechanisms that governed the lives of their ancestors and are still present in the animal world. This means that the issue of emotional neglect must be considered, taking these mechanisms into account, individually and together (Figure 3.2).

Cultural factors that may contribute to emotional neglect in children can largely be related to individualism and prioritising the needs of an individual,

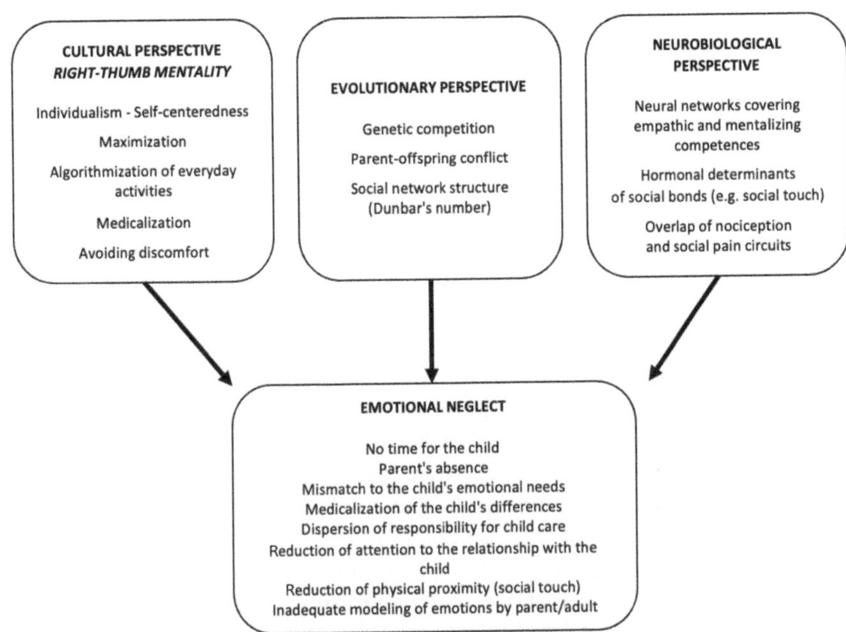

Figure 3.2 Sources of emotional neglect.

such as a parent or caregiver, over the needs of the child. This pertains to the need for comfort and avoiding difficulties. This translates to avoiding touching on issues by the parent (passive and active avoidance/not noticing of difficult topics brought up by the child) and trying to protect the child from experiencing unpleasant emotions. The latter has consequences for the child's disrupted emotional development. Meanwhile, the drive for maximisation leads to the dispersal of caregivers' engagement across many areas of activity, which reduces the possibility of spending time with the child. On the other hand, the desire to provide the child with as many opportunities as possible can translate into a lack of recognising the child's specific needs in favour of scenarios developed by caregivers (and by social demands) and a mismatch between parental activity and the child's needs (lack of interest vs. overabundance). Right-thumb mentality is also associated with the possibility of medicalising the child's problems and potential deviations from the so-called norm adopted in a given society. Thus, it is possible to intensify emotional neglect involving intolerance of individual differences and the unique needs of the child.

Among evolutionary mechanisms, it would be pertinent to mention Dunbar's number, which indicates limitations in expanding the social networks in which we operate. The modern world forces us to create very many contacts and to enter into numerous social interactions, which may lead to a reduction in engagement in close relationships, including the caregiver-child relationship. Familial and neighbourhood connections are also becoming looser, which limits the ability to combine childcare with other members of the closest social group, such as grandparents, neighbours, and uncles/aunts. Thus, an opposite process has occurred compared to that which concerned hominins in the past, where increasing survival chances were linked, among other things, to the development of sharing care for offspring with other group members. The mechanisms related to genetic competition still remain significant. A parent shares only 50% of the genes with a child, leading to an evolutionary conflict of interest in the parent-offspring dyad. Naturally, a parent's investment of resources (including attention) will naturally be dispersed among other already present children or future offspring. It has also been observed that stepfathers have less engagement and a greater tendency for mistreatment of children compared to biological fathers (Alexandre et al., 2010). In the modern world, it can be expected that in blended families, this mechanism of lesser or disrupted engagement of a step-parent may also be present. Genetic competition may also concern siblings, who, wanting to focus parental resources on themselves, may regress to earlier developmental stages in such a way as to capture adult attention.

Inextricably linked to evolutionary mechanisms are neurobiological mechanisms, especially those related to neuronal circuits responsible for processing information about social relationships. Social competencies related to empathy and theory of mind are acquired in relationships with other people in the immediate environment. Meanwhile, modern humans may face problems such as a lack of time for relationships with children, their own inadequate emotional patterns, or lack of frequent contact with children. This will result in inadequate modelling by adults of emotions and disorders in the development of mentalisation by children. Overload, feelings of exclusion, injustice, and relational losses experienced by adults (social pain) can, in turn, lead to the expression of pain witnessed by children. Chronic social pain in individuals with unstable, fragile self-esteem (encouraged by right-thumb social functioning) may translate into emotional numbness, which is another problem in modelling healthy emotionality for a child. Finally, contemporary humans, in fear of violating a child's boundaries and exposing them to sexual abuse, may significantly limit physical closeness between the child and close people. For instance, stepfathers may limit touching children for fear of accusation of sexual abuse. Neighbours or teachers may react similarly. However, social touch theory indicates how important gentle touch is in close relationships for well-being and bond building.

In the following chapters, we will develop a perspective on emotional neglect from cultural, evolutionary, and neurobiological perspectives in an attempt to relate it to the needs of children at various developmental stages.

Chapter 4

Infancy

Being noticed equals surviving

First experiences of full dependence on caregivers

Human evolutionary development has led to a situation where living in larger groups has become possible and brain development has facilitated functioning at a higher level that is inaccessible to other species. The significant increase in brain volume, along with the adoption of an upright posture and bipedal locomotion, necessitated adaptive changes during pregnancy and childbirth. The narrowing of the birth canal in women and the simultaneous increase in the dimensions of the child's head presented a conflict. The evolutionary mechanism of natural selection can be argued to have led to an optimal solution (Brüne, 2016). This is the shortening of gestation time, resulting in the birth of immature infants, which are incapable of independence. Therefore, it could be considered that a human infant is born approximately 13 months prematurely compared with other primates (Jones et al., 1992). On the one hand, this increases the chances of survival for both the child and the mother during childbirth, but on the other hand, it means very long and complete helplessness and dependency of the infant on caregivers. Thus, the child's first developmental task is to survive this period of complete dependence on others, and its key needs are therefore safety and closeness.

The successful establishment of attachment (by the child) and bond (by the parent, usually the mother) is crucial for the child's survival but is also the foundation for the development of a sense of security, self-esteem and the ability to cope with emotions and challenges in the future (Biringen, 2000; Bowlby, 1969; Brüne, 2016; Kim et al., 2017). However, it must be noted that this process requires engagement from both sides of the caregiver-child dyad. From the fourth week of life onwards, babies are increasingly able to engage with caregivers. Infants actively seek contact with their parents, often through crying or laughing, and prefer facial contours to other oval objects and respond to voices, especially the mother's. By the third or fourth month, the infant can distinguish familiar people from strangers and begins to coordinate exchanged visual, vocal, emotional and tactile signals. Positive maternal facial expressions, social gaze, vocalisations and natural olfactory

DOI: 10.4324/9781032621203-4

stimuli have been shown to positively influence inter-brain synchrony in the mother-infant dyad (Endevelt-Shapira & Feldman, 2023).

From around the third month of life, the infant not only develops attachment to the mother but also begins to engage in triadic synchrony, where behaviour is adjusted not only to the interacting parent but also in response to the nonverbal signals exchanged between the parents (Gordon & Feldman, 2008). Parent-infant synchrony, which emerges around the third to fourth month of life, appears to be a critical experience that influences further child development: it promotes the maturation of neuronal circuits involved in processing social and emotional stimuli and fosters the development of a secure attachment style, empathy, self-regulation and the ability to adjust behaviour, as well as future symbolic and moral competencies (Feldman, 2007).

For the mother, seeking closeness with the child is strongly biologically conditioned, but requires active engagement. In mothers, bonding with the child begins during pregnancy when changes occur in the secretion of oxytocin and physiological synchrony between the mother and the child. Oxytocin-assisted bonding continues after childbirth through the breastfeeding process. The physical contact associated with touching and cuddling is also important. Skin-to-skin contact (known as kangarooing) between the caregiver and the child helps regulate stress responses and autonomic functions, improves sleep quality, and supports maturation of the child's prefrontal cortex (Feldman et al., 2014). Tactile stimulation of newborns can prevent some negative behavioural outcomes observed in adulthood including increased susceptibility to substance abuse and increased autistic behaviour in adulthood which may develop as a result of neonatal isolation (Narvaez et al., 2019; Wei et al., 2007). However, establishing a maternal bond often requires support from other adults who can relieve the mother in caregiving and meet her own needs (Hrdy, 2000). This support can come from a partner, other women, friends, relatives and, in modern times, institutions or professional caregivers.

Building attachment – an investment for the future

Understanding infants' innate ability to express basic emotions is crucial for parents and caregivers as it aids in interpreting children's behaviours and appropriately responding to their emotional needs, which is a major factor in preventing emotional neglect. The quality of the emotional bond between parents and child influences the formation of what is termed "attachment style". Introduced by Bowlby (1969), this term describes a state in which an individual feels a strong tendency to seek closeness to another specific individual, referred to as an attachment figure. Once attachment develops in a child, the infant begins to build cognitive and emotional representations of itself and attachment figures. These representations, called "internal working models", determine a child's future approach to exploring the world. Attachment is very stable, and, once formed, it is generally considered irreversible. Human infants can develop more than one attachment, for instance, not only to the mother but also to the father, although these bonds typically have a hierarchical structure. It is worth noting that well-functioning individuals usually have developed attachments to both parents (Hrdy, 2000). Caregivers who are sensitive to the infant's signals and consistently respond to its needs promote the development of secure attachment (Ainsworth et al., 2015). Conversely, inappropriate caregiver responses can lead to the development of insecure attachments (avoidant, ambivalent or disorganised). Attachment style not only affects the infant's relationships with caregivers but also influences its future social interactions and emotional development. Infants with secure attachment typically develop better social skills, exhibit higher self-esteem and are better adapted to stress management (Sroufe et al., 2005). On the other hand, children with insecure attachment may encounter difficulties in building healthy interpersonal relationships and in regulating emotions.

Differences in behaviour and neuro-behavioural functioning associated with attachment styles are primarily shaped by external conditions such as the behaviour of parents or caregivers. The significance of the environment may also have an additional pathway of influence related to gene-environment interactions. It has been shown that reduced activity of MAO-A, associated with a specific polymorphism of the genes encoding (spell out these two) MAO-A and MAO-B, leads to the development of personality disorders and antisocial behaviours (Brüne, 2016). However, this occurs only when children carrying this polymorphism experience violence or neglect in their early life environment. Conversely, friendly and warm conditions can even reduce the risk of antisocial behaviours in these children.

A lack of emotional interaction can lead to "turning off" or apathy (Emde & Easterbrooks, 1985). Studies by Rogol (2020) have shown that infants experiencing emotional deprivation suffer from energy deficiencies. The consequence of disrupted interactions between an infant and its mother or primary caregiver is Maternal Deprivation Syndrome (MDS), which usually appears very early, in infancy. MDS can lead to serious developmental issues for children, both physically and emotionally (Huot et al., 2007; Kalinichev & Francis, 2010). This syndrome is characterised by growth inhibition (failure-to-thrive), feeding problems, emotional disturbances, developmental delays, and changes in brain structures (Čater & Majdič, 2022). Children with MDS may also show reduced interest in their surroundings, apathy, sleep disturbances, and difficulties in forming attachments (Rogol, 2020). The causes of MDS can vary and include factors such as inadequate home conditions, lack of appropriate emotional stimulation, neglect, and mental health issues of the mother or primary caregiver, which prevent the formation of a healthy bond with the child.

To be noticed and welcomed

These considerations clearly highlight the role of emotional interactions between parent and infant in child development, which aligns with various theories describing child emotional development such as Discrete Emotion Theory, Functionalist Theory, Sociocultural Theory, or the Dynamic Systems approach (Hertenstein & Campos, 2001; Fogel et al., 1992; Holodynski, 2009; Lench et al., 2011; Mitsven et al., 2020). Infants, not yet familiar with language, communicate with their environment only through touch and emotions. Studies conducted in the still-face paradigm have repeatedly shown that the liveliness of a parent's facial expressions affects child behaviour and stress. Bornstein et al. (2012) noted that maternal emotional unavailability (still-face paradigm) was more stressful for 4-month-old infants than maternal physical unavailability (separation paradigm). In contrast, research by Sorce and Emde (1981), in which mothers read a newspaper and demonstrated emotional unavailability (despite physical presence), while in another group, mothers were emotionally available, responding sensitively to their children's needs. This showed that children whose mothers were emotionally unavailable exhibited less desire to explore, showed less joy, and spent more time close to their mothers but also sought their attention less frequently.

In today's world, the role of newspapers in Sorce and Emde's (1981) study may be taken by smartphone screens (Braune-Krickau et al., 2021; Khourochvili, 2017; Kildare & Middlemiss, 2017; Myruski et al., 2018). Parents deeply engaged with their smartphones respond less to subtle signals and attempts by their children to interact, show less emotional support, and are less sensitive (Abels et al., 2018; Elias et al., 2020; Vanden Abeele, 2020; Wolfers et al., 2020). This may be related to the right-thumb mentality's need to care for one's own individual needs. In the first year of life, parents are often overwhelmed by responsibilities and have significantly reduced capabilities to satisfy their own needs related to well-being, such as the need for autonomy, relationships and competence (Ryan & Deci, 2000). Using a smartphone while caring for an infant may seem to be a natural way to maintain at least a minimal level of these needs (Chatton, 2017). On the other hand, parents are bombarded with recommendations to be mindful of their infants, which can lead to ambivalence and tension regarding the use of these devices (Braune-Krickau et al., 2021). Creating a secure bond between a child and a parent requires facial emotional expression from parents, which conveys warmth and engagement. However, distraction by smartphone screens can signal a lack of parental engagement and can also be a source of inadequate and incomprehensible emotions in the child (Raudaskoski et al., 2017). Content read from the screen may evoke emotions in parents that have nothing to do with the child-caregiver relationship.

Emotional communication between infant and parent

Inadequate emotional reactions may also be related to difficult relationships between parents, economic problems, and strong stressors that parents experience. The right-thumb tendencies mentioned in Chapter 2, such as maximisation, individualism or discomfort avoidance, may provide additional stressors associated with the frustration of needs. Increasingly, the challenging aspects of parenting are discussed openly, and the right of parents to have time for themselves is being recognised. However, the way these needs are met can sometimes take a dichotomous form: all or nothing. Each of these options can be harmful to the child. A lack of contact intensifies stress in the child, while an excessive search for contact by the parent can lead to a mismatch of parental behaviours with the child's needs. Endevelt-Shapira and Feldman (2023) showed that the synchrony between infant and mother depends on the level of sensitivity or intrusiveness of the mother. Sensitivity included recognising the child's signals, tender eye contact, affection, and gentle touch. Intrusiveness encompasses controlling behaviours, such as excessive stimulation of the child, anxiety, and disregard for the child's pace and rhythm. Greater sensitivity favoured higher synchrony, whereas greater intrusiveness resulted in lower brain-to-brain synchrony between the mother and infant.

The current affective state of a parent can include various emotions, such as anxiety, anger, sadness (including depression), and joy. These emotions are expressed not only in facial expressions but also in the way of speaking. It seems that infants prefer listening to speech known as infant-directed speech (baby talk), characterised by a calm tone, slow pace, emphasised and rising intonation, frequent pauses, and clear pronunciation of simple words, including "babyfied" onomatopoeic words. However, Singh et al. (2002) demonstrated that children prefer listening to happy adult talk over less joyful baby talk. These results suggest that the emotional quality of contact with an infant is more important than mechanical attentiveness. The latter can be undertaken in depressive states or in situations where the parent tries forcibly to conform to educational and media recommendations.

Right-thumb traps in infancy

Sociocultural progress obliges adults to fulfil their parental roles responsibly. As noted in Chapter 2, right-thumb mentality favours solutions based on scientifically supported principles. This is probably why parenting guides and manuals about childcare methods are very popular. On the one hand, this allows inexperienced and/or those without good role models to orient themselves towards good practices. On the other hand, it can be a trap. Let us consider the following examples.

Experiments in the still-face paradigm have shown the importance of emotional expressions in the parent-child relationship. However, if a parent, for some reason, has deficits in the emotional sphere, attempts to purposefully construct emotions within themselves, known as "emotional labour" (Hochschild, 1983), can be difficult and bring opposite effects. Zahn et al. noted that superficial actions related to emotional labour may lead to emotional exhaustion, and more often to negative reactions from partners in the interaction. Translating these results into the parent-infant situation, one can expect increasing frustration on the part of the parent and a lack of the desired effect on the part of the child. The parent may feel impatient, disappointed, and even guilty for not trying hard enough.

The important role of breastfeeding in the development of a bond with the child has been mentioned below. However, there are situations in which breastfeeding is difficult or impossible. On the side of a mother who is strongly attached to the idea of breastfeeding, difficulties with this can lead to feelings of being a bad mother, incomplete motherhood and harming the child may arise. This, in turn, may lead to frustration and the expression of negative emotions, or to an attempt to compensate for the child's excessive care in order to compensate him for this loss. There is a risk of inadequate reading and response to a child's natural needs, and thus neglecting them. A special case may be postpartum depression in the mother. On the one hand, depressive symptoms may be the reason for the mother's inadequate response to the child's needs and may even be associated with a threat to the life of the mother and child through potential suicide. However, the possibility of starting antidepressants by the mother requires weaning the child from breastfeeding. In this case, people who are strongly attached to the idea of breastfeeding may want to reject antidepressant drug therapy. Then breastfeeding is still possible, but emotional contact with the child significantly deteriorates.

Parents can also be overwhelmed by recommendations to actively spend time with their child. However, it is easy to imagine a situation in which a parent (e.g., father) returns home late after a long day of work and wants to engage in interaction and build a bond with the infant. This may lead to the child being bombarded with strong and emotional stimuli that are completely incompatible with biological rhythms and the child's need for sleep and peace. As a result, the child may experience prolonged crying and sleep disturbances. This, in turn, leads to a sense of incompetence and frustration on the part of the well-intentioned parent.

Difficult experiences from a schema modes perspective

Numerous studies and clinical observations suggest that emotional neglect in infants can stem from the negative or traumatic experiences of parents (especially mothers) during their own childhood (Hipwell et al., 2019; Monk et al., 2012; Cort et al., 2011; Wang et al., 2023; Youngblade & Belsky,

1988). As previously mentioned, infants are entirely dependent on their caregivers. Whether caregivers notice and respond to an infant's needs is crucial for survival, and deprivation of these needs can be a source of tension perceived as a life-threatening danger to the child. In prehistoric times, a neglected hominin child died quickly. For helpless infants, the common response to threat is often a "freeze" response, which temporarily allows them to "become invisible" to predators. However, this favours dissociation, understood as a discontinuity or disruption of normally integrated functions, such as consciousness, perception, attention, memory, and identity (DSM-5, 2013; Frewen et al., 2021; Reinders & Veltman, 2021). Dissociation helps coping with mortal fear and unbearable emotions in dangerous situations. It is a highly adaptive strategy; however, if there is no reintegration of experiences after the danger subsides, dissociation can hinder the long-term integration of emotional, cognitive, and sensory processes (Lanius, 2015). Elements of the stressful event become fragmented and are stored in this form to later return as intrusions and retrospections (Spiegel & Cardeña, 1991). For children up to the second year of life, owing to the immaturity of the hippocampus, these fragments are primarily stored as body memories. Again, it should be emphasised that from an evolutionary perspective, a lack of parental attention can be a threatening state for an infant. The result of post-traumatic dissociation will be the formation within the individual's psyche of at least two separately organised systems that cannot be integrated with personality (Peichl, 2007). According to the schema theory by Young et al. (2003), upon activation of a traumatic memory, so-called schema modes may be activated, defined as specific moment-to-moment emotional and behavioural coping states. If a parent has experienced traumatic events resulting in their own schema modes, they may be activated by stimuli from the infant-parent relationship. Parents and infants bring their own vulnerability to injury into this relationship; in the case of the infant, it is evolutionarily conditioned, and in the case of the parent, it depends on their schema modes (Figure 4.1).

Chronic deprivation of a parent's needs can trigger traumatic memories from their own childhood and activate past experiences of childhood fears, anger, or feelings of abandonment. These experiences, echoing the past, can intermingle with current experiences and disrupt the perception of the needs of their real and completely dependent infant. In such cases, there is an inadequate reception and understanding of the signals sent by the child. For example, a child's crying may be associated with the parent's own childhood needs and interpreted as a result of feelings of loneliness and the need for closeness. The activated mode of the "Vulnerable Child" in a parent may respond with attempts at intrusive close contact with the real infant, which on the one hand may be excessive for the child, and on the other, may prevent the identification of the real need signalled by the crying (e.g., hunger, pain, or a full diaper). Conversely, the schema mode of the "Punitive Parent" or "Demanding" or "Critical Parent" may interpret

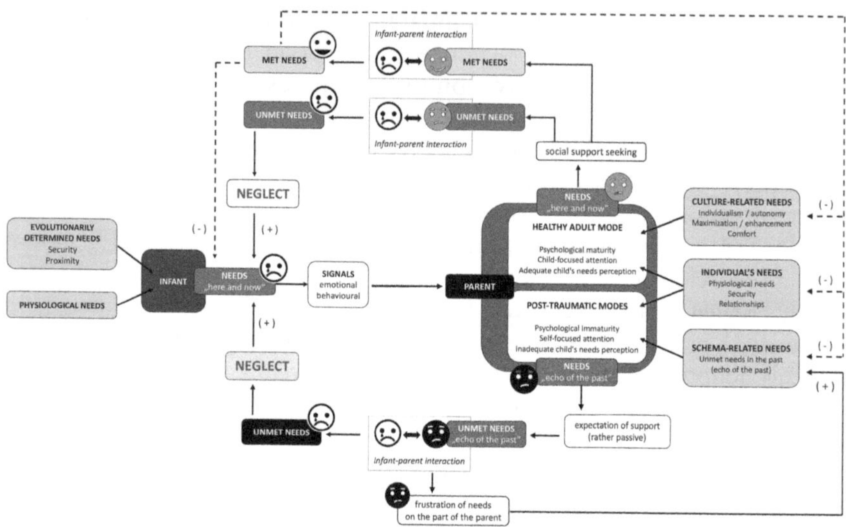

Figure 4.1 Interaction of needs in the infant-parent dyad and child neglect.

the same crying differently. If these modes are directed inward, they can awaken in the parent a sense of guilt and a tendency towards self-sacrifice, and even the development of depressive states (which worsens emotional contact with the infant). However, when these modes are directed outward, there is a tendency to blame others for the child crying, such as the other parent. This leads to tension in the parental dyad, which can be registered by the infant and perceived as a threat.

Activated schema modes in parents must be well recognised and buffered through what's known as the "Healthy Adult" schema mode, which allows for a compromise between the child's needs and the parent's mode needs (child-like needs). The Healthy Adult is capable of consciously delaying gratification and meeting their own needs, tolerates frustration, is empathetic and predictable. While devoting attention to the child, this mode also takes care of itself by ensuring support from close ones. Here again, the issue of taking care of parents' needs arises. The Healthy Adult is a very mature mode, but it is also much weaker than other modes formed in traumatic childhood. If we try to activate the Healthy Adult mode, considering sociocultural changes, we can expect a certain split into two phenomena. The Healthy Adult may be based on natural processes, a collection of intuitive methods developed through mutual observation in the dyad with the child. However, it may also be different. As a result of right-thumb algorithmisation and scientifically sounding advice, this mode may be guided not so much by the natural needs of the child but by media suggestions about "mature parenting". In the latter case, there is a high likelihood of committing emotional neglect with an infant.

In summary, in the infant period, emotional neglect manifests as a mismatch between parents' behaviours and the real emotional needs of the infant, that is, the need for security, attentiveness, and closeness. These needs have their evolutionary and physiological conditions, and satisfying them requires direct emotional contact with the parent in the "here and now". The lack of attention from the parents perceived by the child (their absence in the infant's field of vision, both physically and emotionally; see: still-face paradigm) can be as threatening as excessive care, resulting from the activation of the parent's non-adaptive child-like schemas ("parent's past echoes", leading to emotional absence in the infant-parent interaction) or from caregivers' inadequate understanding of the infant's physiological and developmental needs. Emotional neglect in infancy ultimately leads to the risk of future mental disorders (Braun & Bock, 2011; Norman et al., 2012; Van den Bergh et al., 2006), changes in neuronal function and brain development (Naughton et al., 2013; Roth et al., 2018), changes in social functioning (Lanius, 2015), suicidal behaviours (Felitti et al., 1998), and a decrease in immunity (Jewkes et al., 2010). These consequences significantly interfere with the child's further development.

Chapter 5

Toddlerhood

First steps under the watchful eye of an adult

Intensive toddler brain development

The toddler years, from ages one to three years, are on the one hand a continuation of the dynamic, comprehensive development seen in infancy, and on the other hand, a time for building entirely new competencies: distinguishing oneself as an individual and developing personal autonomy, self-control, expanding one's world and mastering language. All of these factors elevate the child to an entirely new level of functioning. However, similar to infancy, this is a period during which the child is extremely vulnerable, still dependent on caregivers, and susceptible to trauma resulting from neglect, including emotional neglect.

Children's emotional experiences, particularly intense ones, influence the development of neuronal circuits and formation of schemas, especially in the first two years of life (Heim et al., 2010). During this period, most cortical structures undergo rapid development. Traumatic experiences can disrupt this process through the mechanism of epigenetic programming (Lester et al., 2018). It is important to note that memory of events in the early years depends on the maturity of brain structures, such as the amygdala and hippocampus. While the child is born with a mature amygdala, which is responsible for emotional memory, the hippocampal structures, which are responsible for episodic memory, mature later in life. The immaturity of the hippocampus is responsible for so-called childhood amnesia, meaning the inability to form episodic memories until about the age of three years (Lee et al., 2017). Thus, a child's memory mainly consists of context-free emotional and sensory experiences that are processed and stored by the amygdala. Therefore, traumatic experiences are encoded in memory as emotions and somatic sensations. It is possible that flashbacks may occur in the future, triggered by sensory stimuli (e.g., a smell), emotional stimuli (e.g., fear relevant to the current situation that is associated with the fear from a traumatic experience), or somatic triggers (e.g., a specific body position, touch, pain) (Invitto & Grasso, 2019; Vermetten & Lanius, 2012). Thus, a significant challenge for caregivers of toddlers is protecting their children from traumatic experiences. Recall that,

DOI: 10.4324/9781032621203-5

from an evolutionary standpoint, the lack of emotional closeness to a completely dependent child poses a survival threat to toddlers (see Chapter 3). However, staying emotionally close is not the only challenge faced by parents of toddlers.

An open door to emotional neglect

The first signs of the emergence of self-awareness in children typically occur in the second year of life. By then, a child can recognise themselves in a mirror or photograph and understand the concept of ownership (being able to identify objects as their own). This rapid development of autonomy can be exciting, but it is also the source of many tensions and conflicts in the parent-child dyad, which were not present in infancy. Anger develops, shame emerges and the child's curiosity reaches an unimaginable level. One of the most important characteristics of this developmental period is learning through the imitation of adults and older children and confronting newly formed autonomous competencies with social limitations and rules. This necessitates particularly careful development of relationships between parents and toddlers. Let us examine a few examples where issues of emotional neglect might arise and the potential consequences for further development of the child.

As toddlers gain greater independence, the development of their motor skills allows them to expand their world. They are no longer confined to their crib or a small section of the floor. Maintaining an upright position, and increasingly coordinated walking enables them to see and experience more. The natural curiosity inherent in this stage of development drives children to intensively explore their surroundings. What is found in these spaces depends solely on caregivers; children at this age are not yet able to create their own fantastical worlds, so they use and interact with what their caregivers organise in their environment. It falls on the caregivers to ensure that, within the child's reach, there are neither dangerous objects nor items precious to parents. Expecting a child not to touch things important to the parent is a clear mismatch with the developmental norms. Moreover, the plethora of stimuli can be overwhelming, and children may become confused in this new world. They are not yet able to discern many behaviours that may be threatening or inappropriate in their environment. The introduction of rules helps to structure their functioning in this new space of experience. On one hand, rules provide safety by relying on predictability. However, they restrict the emerging autonomy. Czub (2003) has shown that children aged 11–17 months hear prohibitions from their parents every nine minutes on average. However, too many rules do not adequately serve their functions. On the one hand, the child may not be able to master them; on the other hand, for the rules to be effective, the parent needs to be consistent, which can be challenging to maintain. Parents may forget or fail to follow them. Meanwhile, modelling by the parent is key. A lack of good examples from adults can be seen as a type of neglect stemming from a lack of understanding of the developmental stage and needs of the child. Rules that are well suited to the child's developmental capabilities help establish healthy boundaries, which, in turn, are one of the basic emotional needs of children.

At this age, children learn through imitation. They observe adults and replicate their behaviours. At this stage, colourful toys become less significant, while "pretend play" of adult activities gains importance. Cooking, cleaning, reading or engaging in any activity becomes infinitely more interesting, simply because an adult significant to the child is involved. The actual meaning of the activity is secondary. The result of the activity is also irrelevant; the child focuses on the process itself and repeats it multiple times. Here, the role of the adult is to patiently accompany the child and demonstrate each action repeatedly. Attempts to do things for children are counterproductive. For example, when a child is doing something slowly, the desire to help can instil a sense of failure to meet expectations and a sense of shame, which will be discussed later in this chapter.

Language – a new form of communication

Between the ages of one and three years, a child's language abilities develop intensively. The more extensive the child's vocabulary, the easier it becomes for them to navigate the social world, increasing their future chances of success in various fields (Avila-Varela et al., 2021; Morgan et al., 2015; Rantalainen et al., 2021). The influence of the environment is crucial for vocabulary acquisition, specifically, what linguistic stimuli reach the child and from whom (e.g., adults, other children, media) (Fitch et al., 2020). The role of the environment in language development is emphasised in all models of language acquisition and is consistent across cultures. The amount and quality of linguistic input from caregivers are equally significant to the rate of vocabulary acquisition (Head Zauche et al., 2016). The way families use media is described as family media ecology (Linebarger & Vaala, 2010), where cultural influences that families identify with and the associated beliefs, behaviour patterns and values play a crucial role (Acerbi, 2016).

It is important to consider situations in which immigrant families might also want to use media to support language learning for their children (and themselves) (e.g., Cycyk & Hammer, 2020). While some studies have shown a positive impact of media on language development, others have observed the opposite effect (Cycyk & De Anda, 2021). The factor that seems to explain these discrepancies is the involvement of caregivers. According to the socio-pragmatic approach to language development, it is assumed that children, by actively interacting with more linguistically competent individuals (here: parents, caregivers), learn meanings from them, and through practising newly acquired words and language structures in interactions, learn language more quickly (Lavigne et al., 2015; Mendelsohn et al., 2010; Tomasello, 2000).

Children using media without active caregiver involvement does not support their development (Nathanson & Rasmussen, 2011). Parents tend to speak less to their child when the television is on, even when it is just in the background, and not only when watching it is the main activity (Anderson & Hanson, 2017). This is particularly significant considering that in nearly 60% of households, TV is on, even though no one is watching it (Zoromba et al., 2023). Simply having children watch programmes intended for adults does not support their language development (Barr et al., 2010). Furthermore, Christakis et al. (2009) found that each hour a child spends in front of television is associated with a reduction of 770 words spoken to the child by the parents.

The way parents speak to their children also matters. Specialised child-directed speech, by emphasising words, varying tone, adjusting pace, repeating phrases, and supporting statements with questions, helps children absorb new words and language structures (Kidd & Rowland, 2021; Longobardi et al., 2016; Zauche et al., 2016). However, this type of speech must be adapted to the increasing language abilities of children, which requires a high degree of attentiveness from adults. This can be particularly challenging when an adult interacts with a larger group of children, such as in day care centres or nurseries. In these instances, the educational and relational skills of caregivers play a crucial role (Kidd & Rowland, 2021), and these skills can often be insufficient (Hindman et al., 2021; LaParo et al., 2009).

Media as an opportunity and risk for toddlers' development

The presence of media in the lives of toddlers is not only a matter of supporting their language development. In the previous chapter, we addressed the issue of infants' parents using smartphones, which can fall into the still-face paradigm and send emotionally inadequate signals to infants. This phenomenon continues to be highly relevant for toddlers. Children are unable to discern the real emotional disposition of a parent, and their stage of cognitive development does not allow them to guess their parental intentions. The facial expressions sent by the parents are taken literally. Raudaskoski et al. (2017) referring to these phenomena with the concept of "bystander ignorance", point out that the parent's shift of attention to a screen significantly impairs the possibility of mutual attention exchange and eye contact between the parent and child, as well as the child's ability to learn through imitation. At most, parent models engaged with a smartphone are extremely important activities, as this can lead to problematic use of smartphones and media by children in the future. However, some aspects of media use can have a beneficial impact on maintaining close bonds with absent parents or relatives (McClure, 2017).

For toddlers, the use of digital devices also includes a novel phenomenon. This involves using media and digital devices to occupy children or soothe their difficult emotions (Coyne et al., 2021). There has long been a growing problem with young children using media, with the vast majority (75–96%) using them daily (Mack, 2012; Rideout, 2017; Zoromba et al., 2023), spending an average of about an hour to over three hours per day in front of screens (Rideout, 2017; Zoromba et al., 2023), and 92.2% of children using media before they turn one year old (Zoromba et al., 2023). Moreover, the WHO (2019) recommends that preschool children's screen time should not exceed one hour per day.

Children most commonly watch cartoons or engage in games, and, as Zoromba et al. (2023) show, only about 2.3% of children watch educational programmes. Importantly, the same studies note that only approximately 26% of parents always monitor what their child is watching, and 37% of parents are either completely or insufficiently aware of what their child is watching or playing. Kabali et al. (2015) showed that most children primarily watched Netflix or YouTube. This observation is significant because these platforms offer the possibility of viewing content in loops and sequences that do not require mechanical switching; hence, parent interventions are not required for extended periods. It seems that the media serve the function of occupying children, while parents can attend to their own matters. Given parents' permanent lack of time for themselves and the need to balance many tasks (right-thumb maximisation), it is not surprising that the tendency to provide children with media is increasing (Goode et al., 2019). Parents may justify their decisions by wanting to expand their children's horizons through media, assuming the positive impact of media on vocabulary development, and so on. However, considering that many parents do not know what their children are watching and the numerous reports of children developing slower when spending more time in front of screens, this seems to be mainly an illusion that calms parental anxiety. It is worth recalling observations by Levine et al. (2019), who noted the particularly negative effects on children who use media without parental supervision.

Another important function of media is to soothe toddlers' difficult emotions (Radesky et al., 2016; Zoromba et al., 2023). Media can effectively divert attention and regulate emotions, which is described as media emotion regulation (Radesky et al., 2016). However, it is important to remember that the post-infancy period is crucial for the development of emotional self-regulation (Shin & Kemps, 2020). Soothing difficult affective experiences through the media disrupts this process and seems to be a risky strategy because of the potential for developing unhealthy affect regulation patterns (Gordon-Hacker & Gueron-Sela, 2020). However, the benefits of using the potential of negative emotions may usually appear in the distant future, whereas the soothing effect of using the media is immediate. This mechanism strongly reinforces the use of media by both the children and their parents.

Emotional development in contact with others

In terms of psychosocial development in children aged 12–16 months, further development of attachment (Deneault et al., 2023), theory of mind (Ruffman, 2023), and empathy (Paulus et al., 2024) is observed; they begin to self-regulate their emotions and start interacting with peers (Wesarg-Menzel et al., 2023). These are specific milestones whose achievements have significant implications for the child's future. Deviations in these areas can lead to serious developmental difficulties and severe functional disorders in the future.

In the emotional development of toddlers, new emotions (such as shame or pride) and nuances of emotions (such as embarrassment and intimidation) appear. The increasing complexity of emotional experiences also enables a better understanding of what is happening in other people. It is during this period that empathy and mentalisation intensively develop.

For the development of empathy and theory of mind, which allow a toddler to acquire the ability to recognise the mental state of others, relationships with parents are very important. Compared to children with a secure attachment style, those who develop an insecure attachment style are slower to develop the ability to mentalise (Althoff, 2023). It has been observed that children whose parents talk to them about emotions and comment on "emotional" experiences (including relational ones) develop better empathy and mentalisation (Dollberg & Hanetz-Gamliel, 2023). Interestingly, Meins et al. (2002) noted that maternal mind-mindedness, which is the mother's awareness of the child's mind, and thereby treating it as an entity with its own distinct, unique mind, facilitates the building of attachment and theory of mind in the child.

The development of empathy begins in infancy (Hoffman, 2008). By the end of the first year of life, children show egocentric empathy; for example, when hearing another child crying, they themselves cuddle up to their mother. In the second year of life, pseudo-egocentric empathy appears; that is, the child reacts to another person's suffering by wanting to help them. However, this help takes forms that are soothing for the child itself (e.g., they comfort another person by giving them their favourite toy). From around the 18th month of life, or rather from the moment of a clearer perception of the separateness of one's own self, the development of proper empathy begins, and will continue to develop throughout life.

Children learn to name and regulate emotions through contact with more experienced models, most often with their closest people (Fields-Olivieri et al., 2020; Kopp, 1989). They learn by watching adults and what adults do, not what they say (Oláh & Király, 2019). Observing adults' emotions allows children to understand what is important and how to react to it. Time spent together and the exchange of emotions between children and adults, combined with a discussion of shared experiences, promotes the better use of emotions in the future, as illustrated in Figure 5.1.

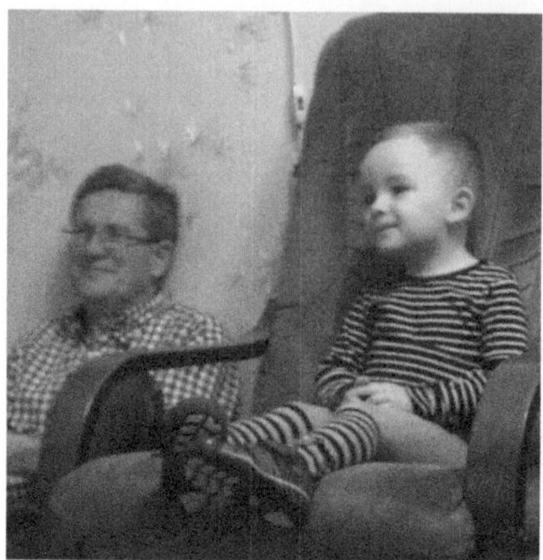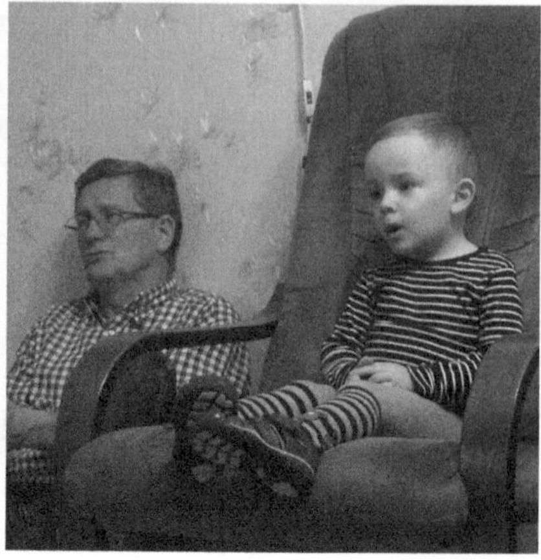

Figure 5.1 Shared emotional experiences between a toddler and caregiver (photograph by Ewa Wojtyna/author's own archive).

However, interactions with children are not always easy. Emerging autonomy contributes to the development of emotions such as anger. Tantrums and the expression of negative emotions peak around the age of two, often referred to as the "terrible twos" (Barry & Kochanska, 2010). Anger can lead to episodes of aggression that sporadically occur in nearly all children aged two and three (Alink et al., 2006). Managing this anger requires significant parental effort. The skilful handling of anger is crucial for establishing healthy boundaries. Therefore, suppressing anger in all situations (e.g. expecting the child to always behave) can be just as harmful as permissive parenting, where the parent allows the child to express anger without limits.

Tantrums may also arise as children develop a sense of ownership in their second year of life, introducing new challenges in the parent-child dyad. Parents wanting to encourage their child's prosocial behaviours or to boast about their "good upbringing" might force the child to share toys with other children. Suddenly, the child may refuse to do so, although this is not a problem during infancy. For the child, sharing toys may be unacceptable and incomprehensible. Forcing a child into such a behaviour could be seen as an infringement, overstepping boundaries, and the emotional stance of the parent may lead to shaming the toddler. In turn, shame can inhibit future prosocial behaviours in children.

A similar misunderstanding of ownership can occur when discarding the various items to which the child is attached. As children's exploration of the world and curiosity grow, they may collect various objects (pebbles, feathers, sticks, glass shards, etc.). The parent, aiming to ensure cleanliness in the child's room, might want to remove such collections, not understanding that they may represent invaluable treasures to the child.

During the post-infant period, toddlers develop new types of self-conscious emotions (Tracy & Robins, 2007). One of the key emotions here is shame, which arises when an individual perceives that they have violated a norm considered important. This results in a painful, intense feeling accompanied by beliefs of worthlessness, flaws, evil, or deserving of contempt. Behavioural indicators such as slumped posture, head down, blushing, and hiding the face accompany this emotion. These behaviours have deep evolutionary significance—they help restore proper social status and protect one's safety from the group's anger (Gilbert, 1997).

However, misuse by adults of the ability to induce shame in children, as well as adult reactions to a child's shame, are crucial areas for reflection on emotional neglect. Parents who are eager to demonstrate their parenting competencies to society (where a child's behaviour is an objective indicator that can be interpreted through a right-thumb black-and-white unambiguity) may experience unnecessary tension when the child's behaviour deviates from that desired. A parent experiencing their own shame or disappointment due to their child's behaviour may react aggressively, punish silently, or clearly show their disappointment, inducing shame in the child. As a result, the child may fear engaging in further activities in an area that displeases the parent. The child might stop expressing autonomy and desire to act. This parental behaviour aligns with the schema-based approach described in Chapter 4 (Young et al., 2003). Activation of schema modes (e.g., the Vulnerable or Angry Child mode) can make soothing parents' own negative affect more important than patiently accompanying the child. It is crucial for parents to understand their psychological state and be aware of potential post-traumatic disorders and other mental health issues.

This issue is particularly evident in the child-parent dyad, where a parent suffers from Post-traumatic Stress Disorder (PTSD). Although a child's outburst of anger does not pose a significant real threat, it may be associated with the parent's traumatic experiences. Studies have shown that PTSD contributes to responding with negative affect to emotionally charged situations (Orsillo et al., 2004), and heightened negative emotions lead to less effective parenting behaviours (Rueger et al., 2011). For a parent with PTSD or Complex Post-traumatic Stress Disorder (cPTSD) not only the situational context (the parent must handle the difficult task of managing child noncompliance), but also the emotion itself can trigger flashbacks and emotional experiences, which are intrusions from the past. This activates the parent's stress response system. In post-traumatic disorders, two stress response patterns typically develop (Del Giudice et al., 2011). The first pattern involves hypervigilance associated with increased stress reactivity and enhanced negative affect, which can lead to an increase in negative-intrusive parental behaviours during play with children (Mills-Koonce et al., 2009). The second pattern involves a reduction in physiological and affective responses to stress, which manifests as diminished emotional expression (Juul et al., 2015). Each of these patterns predisposes children to an inadequate response to their anger. Post-traumatic attention distortions in a parent lead to a cascade of further cognitive distortions and negative emotions associated with parenthood, worsening the relationship with the child (Creech & Misca, 2017). To reduce the risk of triggering strong negative emotions when confronted with a child's anger, a parent might engage in overly harsh behaviours (attempting to quickly suppress the child's undesirable behaviour) or overly indulgent behaviours (trying to calm the child's negative affect and seeking peace) (Lorber & O'Leary, 2005). More frequent engagement in a permissive parenting pattern has been observed among mothers who exhibit partial PTSD symptoms (Franz et al., 2022). These findings support the observations that individuals with traumatic experiences, due to their intolerance of negative affect, more often resort to strategies that allow avoidance of discomfort and adopt permissive behaviours to achieve greater peace.

Excessive concern for children's development

In toddlers, there are significant variations in the rate of development, which can affect many parents. Comparisons with other children through seeking information in the media and parenting guides can lead to steps towards diagnosing various issues and implementing various developmental support methods. Early identification of serious problems allows for very early specialist interventions that can protect the child from debilitating future consequences. Consider one example: the early diagnosis of autistic spectrum disorders (ASD).

ASD can be diagnosed relatively early, between the ages of 18 and 24 months. This enables the initiation of interventions that can effectively improve the child's cognitive, communicative, social, and motor functioning (Okoye et al., 2023; Taylor et al., 2015; Vivanti et al., 2014), which also helps reduce the overall long-term care costs (Järbrink & Knapp, 2001). Such early intervention can also be beneficial for the entire family by increasing access to support and reducing parental stress (Grzadzinski et al., 2021). Although early diagnosis is undoubtedly helpful, it carries several risks including overdiagnosis and overtreatment (Howes et al., 2018; Okoye et al., 2023). These risks are greatest in the youngest children, as the clinical picture of ASD is limited in specificity and the diagnostic process may lead to false-positive results (Guthrie et al., 2013). Children often exhibit some symptoms that are not strong enough to meet the criteria for ASD diagnosis. Nevertheless, it is observed that such children often receive specialised treatment, such as pharmacotherapy or behavioural therapy (Brookman-Frazee et al., 2018; Paris, 2015). Medications and behavioural therapy can have different effects from those intended. The side effects of pharmacological treatment can outweigh the expected benefits; hence, drugs are recommended as supportive treatments rather than for routine use (Howes et al., 2018). Nevertheless, there is a risk that the desire to quickly achieve an effect by eliminating at least some symptoms (right-thumb tendencies) will lead to these drugs being used more often than is actually indicated. Meanwhile, behavioural therapy (applied behaviour analysis), despite many robust studies of its effectiveness, is becoming increasingly controversial, especially among autism rights and neurodiversity activists, who point out the risk of abuse against children (Leaf et al., 2022). Therefore, early implementation of treatment requires serious critical analysis and, if indications for therapy are maintained, finding a safe way to conduct it, which may often be too difficult for parents (Bickel et al., 2015). From another perspective, experiences of stigmatisation associated with ASD diagnoses have also been noted (Rotholz et al., 2017). Finally, diagnostic and therapeutic procedures are time consuming. For parents who already have little of it, there may be a lack of space for everyday ordinary time spent together and the building of child-parent relationships.

Summarising the considerations above, the biggest challenge for the post-infant period seems to be parents helping children develop a compromise between the desire for autonomy and the need to conform to social norms. It is crucial for adults to participate actively in these processes. It has been shown that an unmet need in a child for direct closeness with an adult (parent, caregiver) increases the tendency to seek contact with an adult, and this tendency dominates the need to explore the world (Ali et al., 2021). This hinders the development of a child's autonomy in favour of meeting social environmental expectations. Considering that it is during this developmental period that the foundations for future personality are laid, this phenomenon is of special significance. An additional emotionally significant process is the neglect by adults of the child's needs (due to ignorance of developmental processes or culturally imposed directions, such as unambiguity or maximisation) that can disturb children's previously developed sense of trust in the world. This translates into a child turning away from a reality that only means frustration. Excessive control by adults, by inducing a sense of shame in the child, can destroy their curiosity and spontaneity. Conversely, an insufficient level of control, resulting in a lack of boundaries, can inhibit children's activity because of their growing sense of anxiety. The most important conclusion from reflections on the post-infant stage is thus the necessity for engaged adult participation in children's attempts to take their first steps, not only physically, but also in terms of asserting their own autonomy and exploring an ever-wider world.

Chapter 6

Early childhood

First experiences beyond the boundaries of the home

Going out into the world outside the home

The preschool period, spanning ages three to six years, is a time of gaining independence and a phase of transition from family life to participation in an open, non-domestic environment. The primary developmental task during this period is to reconcile two conflicting tendencies: setting personal goals, and pursuing them in one's own way, while respecting social norms and rules in the environment. In practice, this means children achieving emotional and social readiness to spend several hours a day away from their family environment. Pre-schoolers also undertake activities necessary to learn about different social roles and deepen their self-awareness (Matejczuk, 2014). This chapter examines the factors necessary to achieve developmental goals for preschool-aged children through the lens of potential risks of emotional neglect.

Venturing outside the home environment is an important milestone for children's social and emotional development. For a child to develop curiosity about the outside world and the desire to explore it, the need for security and closeness at home must first be met (Ali et al., 2021). If a child knows that the home is safe and predictable, they can leave it without fear, knowing that it will remain the same upon their return. However, if the home environment is unstable, for example, with parents displaying inconsistent and unpredictable behaviours, the child may not know who will be at home or what the home will look like upon their return. In such cases, a child may be reluctant to leave home, preferring to stay in and continuously monitor the home situation and avoid exploring the external world. Parents must be aware of their children's need for stability. However, if they lead irregular lives themselves – frequently moving, working shifts, or often traveling – such functioning, which is increasingly common in today's sociocultural situation, will not provide that sense of stability. Instability may also stem from conflicts between parents or household members, including domestic violence or substance abuse. Living with a substance-dependent parent under one roof is not uncommon; for instance, Lipari and Van Horn (2017) indicated that

DOI: 10.4324/9781032621203-6

nearly one in eight children in the United States live with a parent who is addicted to psychoactive substances. In addition, a common issue today is that children are raised in single-parent families, where providing a stable home environment is a significant challenge for parents who share custody.

Exploring environments beyond home involves encountering phenomena previously unknown to children. In earlier developmental stages, the child forms a representation of home that is somewhat predictable, uncomplicated, and stable. Beyond this environment, the child must confront the fact that behavioural patterns developed at home no longer work effectively or yield the expected results. This leads to numerous inappropriate, ineffective, and socially unacceptable behaviours that can evoke strong emotional tension in children. Subtle and gentle support from parents, who represent the order of the home and are simultaneously experts in navigating the outside world, is crucial to this transition.

Misunderstanding the developmental stage of a child can cause a parent, upon observing the child's inappropriate behaviours outside the home, to try to suppress them reflexively and harshly. In such situations, a sense of guilt may develop in the child, thereby inhibiting further activities. This is particularly evident among children with insecure attachment styles (Lawrence et al., 2019). Such children tend to experience inappropriate feelings of guilt: this emotion arises too early, often before the child has acted, and is excessively strong, leading to self-restriction, where fear of feeling guilty is a primary mechanism. In contrast to the parental behaviour described above, this approach is based on attentive and healthy controls. When a parent notices that a child is struggling or behaving inappropriately, they model the appropriate behaviour for the child. Important aspects of this modelling process include the parent's attempts to understand the child's intentions, analyse what went wrong, and suggest more effective solutions. This process teaches the child to manage situations through an algorithm: problem – question – reflection – behaviour. However, such learning requires the physical and emotional presence of the parents. Only then can the parent promptly respond to the pre-schooler's problematic behaviours and arrange educational situations in which they can explore the best solutions with the child.

The presence of a parent is crucial. If physical (e.g., trips, long work hours, separations) or psychological distance (e.g., parental mental health issues, lack of interest in the child, online work, or excessive media engagement) grows between the child and the parent, the child will turn to other available sources for behavioural models. Often, they may be older children or peers. Children model behaviour based on the path of least resistance, which means satisfying their needs as quickly as possible. This approach means that children may not learn to balance their desires with social norms, which can lead to the reinforcement of problematic social behaviours and behavioural disorders in the future (Mphaphuli, 2023).

Patient accompaniment

Preschool-aged children have increasingly well-developed memories and start to create narrative memories, although this function has not yet been fully developed. Therefore, children may struggle with generalisation and may not learn from mistakes effectively. This means that, even after parental intervention, children might repeatedly return to inappropriate behaviours. This requires parents to explain and accompany the child repeatedly and patiently.

Another challenging aspect for parents is understanding the variability in their pre-schoolers' desires. When pre-schoolers want something (which happens frequently) but cannot get it immediately, they begin to imagine it. The longer something is unavailable, the more detached these images become from reality. Consequently, the child begins to desire what is in their fantasy. When a child eventually receives the desired object, it often falls short of expectations, leading to disappointment and quick abandonment of the item. This can be extremely frustrating for parents, especially when acquiring the desired toy is not easy (e.g., due to the family's financial situation). Media and advertisements can significantly amplify children's desires (Šramová, 2015). A lack of understanding of this developmental rule can lead parents to interpret the child's behaviour as disrespectful, creating tension and even anger and aggression towards the child. In such cases, the child may either internalise aggressive reactions or withdraw from expressing their needs to the parent (Wilson, 2008).

Parent as a model of behaviour and rules

During the preschool years, children develop moral intuition. Influenced by the commands and prohibitions set by parents, they modify their behaviour either to avoid punishment or, in the case of slightly older children, to gain rewards. However, in each case, children try to obey parents whom they respect. This one-directional respect forms the basis of the characteristic preschool-age morality, known as "heteronomous morality", which is based on complete obedience and a literal approach to the rules imposed on the child (Sengsavang et al., 2015; Smetana, 1981). The child uncritically adopts their caregivers' worldview and enacts the behavioural patterns provided by them. This situation can lead to potential abuse by parents. If a parent imposes too many rules (e.g., to satisfy their own ambitions), introduces rules while joking with the child, or sets rules that are not adapted to the child's capabilities, the child may treat these rules as absolute and assume that no deviations are allowed. This will lead to inappropriate behaviours and expose the child to further conflicts with the parent (because it is impossible to fulfil all rules literally) and with others. Failure to meet these rigid and irrevocable rules can be too challenging for the child and can lead to unbearable tensions. In such cases, the child may experience dissociation (Nijenhuis & van der

Hart, 2011). Other very serious consequences may include the emergence of the need for self-punishment. For preschool-aged children, a literal approach to rules means that the severity of the punishment should be linked to the severity of the transgression (known as "retributive punishment"). If parental neglect occurs at this stage, the child may take actions that have tragic consequences, including suicidal behaviours.

By introducing rules, a parent might be guided by seemingly good intentions. For example, if a parent concerned with maintaining a fit physique and healthy diet loudly repeats that "one must have a flat stomach", the child might take this rule literally. However, a child's physique is not suitable to meet this standard. The child may feel guilty for not adhering to this rule. Their continually protruding belly reminds them of their inadequacy and failure to meet parents' standards. Emotional tension builds in children. It may happen that the child discovers on their own or through imitation that not eating (anorexia) helps achieve a flat stomach in line with the rules while also reducing unpleasant emotional tension (Martin & Strodl, 2023).

The above considerations clearly indicate the parent's role as a behavioural model for the child. It is important that at least one caregiver serves as a role model for the child to identify with. Preschool children mimic their parents and see them as authorities. Thus, they strive towards what is important to the parent, and unconsciously absorb the adult's behavioural patterns. Therefore, parents' actions in various roles must be recognisable, understandable and adoptable by the child. This is not possible if the parent is unavailable, emotionally unstable, or is under the influence of psychoactive substances. A parent's understanding of this mechanism will allow the building of a healthy foundation for the child's independent actions. It is crucial to model positive health-promoting habits, emotional regulation, and conflict resolution. This requires parents to gain insight into their own emotional functioning. Only then will socialisation with emotions proceed correctly in the child. Pre-schoolers experience an increasing range of emotions, yet the way they think about emotions and the behaviours they adopt (i.e., emotional schemas) are modelled by adults (Dennis & Kelemen, 2009).

Increasing understanding of emotions and development of theory of mind

During the preschool stage, there is also significant development in the theory of mind (mentalisation), as discussed in Chapter 3. By the fourth year of life, a child can already construct a representational model of the mind, and by the fifth year, children develop the ability to differentiate real events from thoughts about them. They understand that different people may have different opinions about the same event. They begin to distinguish truth from falsehood and understand what lies or metaphors are. The processes occurring in another person's mind are unobservable; therefore, they can only be inferred based on facial expressions, gestures, speech, behaviour, and experiences from social interactions and self-awareness of one's own mental states (introspection). Having the ability to mentalise is foundational for adaptive social behaviours, as it allows understanding and predicting the behaviour of others. It also enables actions depending on the situation and others' expectations, understanding social norms, manipulating others, understanding punchlines in jokes, and possessing an adaptive sense of humour, which we discuss in Chapter 7.

Both emotional and physical neglect in childhood are associated with improper processing of emotions on faces and face perception (Jin et al., 2023; Neil et al., 2022). Children raised in institutions are less sensitive to happy faces and require more information to distinguish them from neutral faces than children raised in families (Moulson et al., 2015). Research conducted by Ke et al. (2022) suggests that the ability to recognise more complex emotions based on body movements begins to develop around the sixth year of life but is not yet fully mature at this stage of a child's development. Between the ages of 4 and 6 years, children gradually respond better to subtle changes in biological movements, and this sensitivity improves until adolescence. However, processing this type of information requires an environment in which a child can acquire experiences, meaning that interactions with emotionally well-functioning others are necessary. The isolation of the child will favour disturbances in emotional and social functioning (Marryat et al., 2014).

Disturbed identification of feelings (one's own and others'), impaired distinction between physiological and emotional arousal of the body, restricted imagination, and externally oriented thinking (focused on the environment instead of one's own feelings and thoughts) are symptoms of a phenomenon known as alexithymia (Kajanoja et al., 2021; Mikolajczyk & Luminet, 2006). Numerous studies have demonstrated a link between alexithymia and emotional neglect (Aust et al., 2013; Kajanoja et al., 2021; Lumley et al., 2007). Alexithymia is believed to result from inadequate parental bonding and emotional neglect in childhood. This can lead to an insecure attachment style and difficulties in regulating emotions (Lyvers et al., 2019). Research conducted by Aust et al. (2013), showed a significant correlation between the degree of alexithymia and experiences of emotional neglect in early childhood. This is particularly important because other manifestations of childhood trauma, such as physical or sexual violence, did not show a significant association with alexithymia in their study sample.

Although alexithymia can significantly hinder the development of close relationships with others, trust distinctly facilitates this. Brown (2023) referenced several definitions of trust in a literature review. For instance, Allum et al. (2010) define it as an "abstract social value". Nikolakis and Nelson (2019) refer to it as "social glue", and Fukuyama (1995, p. 153) observes that "trust arises when a community shares a set of moral values in such a way as to create expectations of regular and honest behaviour". Regardless of the definition, trust is considered a crucial element in the personal, social, and intellectual development of children (Bernath & Feshbach, 1995). Trust is built from the earliest years of life through interactions with parents and caregivers, and its development is closely linked to a child's experiences. The stability and predictability of the parent are necessary. According to psychological theories, such as Bowlby's attachment theory, which we have mentioned in previous chapters, secure attachment that develops from consistent and caring caregiving is key to building trust. Children need people they can trust, yet studies show that negative childhood experiences have been associated with less trust (Gobin & Freyd, 2014) and "a reticence to trust unfamiliar others" (Neil et al., 2022, p. 656). Individuals who have negative childhood experiences are less likely to exhibit high levels of trust in various types of relationships (Brown, 2023). Meanwhile, children in institutional care settings are less likely to trust their peers and quickly withdraw trust if betrayed by another child (Pitula et al., 2016). Additionally, research by Huang et al. (2022) examining how different parenting styles in the family and their impact on emotional and behavioural problems in preschool children (ages 3–6), considering gender differences, showed that emotional and behavioural problems were more common in children raised in overprotective, laissez-faire, autocratic, and inconsistent styles. Conversely, children raised in democratic parenting styles had significantly fewer such issues. Moreover, boys were more susceptible to the negative effects of overprotective parenting than girls were.

Learning boundaries and rules through play

As indicated above, neither permissive nor restrictive parenting styles foster emotional development. However, building a healthy compromise between children's desires and societal norms is challenging. A preschool-aged child will naturally seek to obtain the desired objects through the path of least resistance. However, when parents perceive potential risks in such spontaneous child behaviours, they often impose limitations. Optimal conditions for setting these limits involve a scenario in which the child loves and respects the boundary-setting parent, who, in turn, teaches the child how to satisfy their needs safely. This guidance can often be delivered effectively through play. By role-playing in various scenarios, children can empathise with the consequences of their actions and attempt to independently decide whether a behaviour is acceptable. Such play should occur under the discreet supervision of parents or caregivers ready to intervene if it takes a dangerous turn. Allowing children to engage in certain types of play requires assurance from parents that the child understands the real-world consequences of forbidden actions such as shooting characters in a game. Preschool children, driven by strong desires, attempt to try new things that may not always be feasible in reality. Here, play aids in learning, as through imaginative identification, children can experience the consequences of different behaviours (e.g. after playing the role of a thief during play who ends up behind bars and experiences the loss of free participation in life).

Facilitating realistic play and role-experimentation opportunities is a crucial task for parents to organise the space in which their children function. If parents structure this space without allowing room for spontaneous activities, children may struggle to develop both social competencies and the foundations of self-esteem. An excess of tightly scheduled extracurricular activities, operating according to pre-determined scripts, gives children illusory choices that often lead to helplessness and loss of spontaneity (Marsh & Kleitman, 2002). Meanwhile, spontaneously initiated play allows children to express their desires, fears, and anxieties and to communicate with their environment (Cooper, 2006; Ginsburg, 2007; Kourkouta & Papathanassiou, 2014), strengthening their communicative, sensorimotor, and creative skills (Parham & Primeau, 1997; Rubin et al., 1983; Russ, 2007; Rye, 2008). Failing to allow children the freedom of spontaneous play is a serious neglect. Conversely, children who have experienced emotional neglect or emotional abuse from their parents often show difficulties in engaging in play (Koenig et al., 2000).

Restricting a child's opportunity for spontaneous expression can also stem from external factors independent of the parent. In such cases, parents' sensitive presence and attunement to their child's emotional needs become crucial. An example of this could be a child's chronic illness (e.g., diabetes) or a condition requiring intensive medical procedures, such as hospitalisations or burdensome treatments (e.g., for oncological patients). These children may be forced to strictly adhere to medical regimes, which can be both incomprehensible and unpleasant. Additionally, their ability to meet their own needs is limited, leading to a reduction in the intensity of these needs and the associated emotional expression (Alamiri et al., 2023; Zheng et al., 2023). To counteract the potential developmental disturbances arising from these conditions, a high degree of parental or caregiver emotional sensitivity is required.

Considering emotional neglect and its impact on pre-schoolers' language abilities (Naughton et al., 2013). Allen and Oliver (1982) found that neglected children (including emotional neglect) showed signs of developmental delay, especially in language skills, compared with physically abused children and a control group. This delay can be observed in both receptive language (understanding from listening) and expressive language (verbal abilities) (Culp et al., 1991). Neglected children struggle with language development because they lack the necessary trust in their environment to feel comfortable speaking. Fear of judgement and shame lead to a lack of speaking practice and ultimately delay their language abilities. Franz et al. (2013) demonstrated that up to 7.5% of pre-schoolers show symptoms of social phobia. Significant insights come from research that considers the types of violence against children. It has been shown that children who experience only neglect may have poorer outcomes in language development and vocabulary range than children who experience both neglect and physical abuse (Allen & Oliver, 1982). This suggests that emotional neglect alone may have deeper or more harmful consequences on cognitive development than a combination of neglect and physical violence.

In summary, neglecting children negatively affects their early development, which can translate into learning difficulties and challenges in adapting to preschool and the first grade through weakened cognitive development (Manly et al., 2013). Neglected children in preschool have more difficulty understanding tasks set by teachers than children who were not neglected. Studies conducted by Manly et al. (2013) among preschool-aged children showed that those who had experienced neglect often had difficulties in preschool, such as in trouble performing tasks and controlling behaviour. In preschool, they also faced greater challenges, and transitioning to the first grade they often received lower grades. Additionally, poor adjustment in preschool due to neglect is a harbinger of cognitive performance difficulties. According to teachers, these children are less engaged in mathematics and language arts, poorly control their behaviour, and have difficulties in social interactions with peers. Meanwhile, considering parental mechanisms of emotional neglect, the neglect of preschool-aged children primarily results from a lack of physical and emotional availability of the parent and a lack of adequate modelling of healthy expression of needs, emotions, and desires, thus failing to build healthy competencies in relationships with people (children and other adults) outside the family system.

Chapter 7

Middle childhood

Opening or closing opportunities for self-development

Challenges in the world of education

Developmental psychology defines the period between 6 or 7 and 12 years as middle childhood (Bogin, 2003; Collins, 1984). During this period, children develop key emotional, cognitive, and social skills that are essential for their future functioning in society. White (1996, p. 17) describes this as the "entry into the age of reasoning". This stage is notable for significant changes in a child's development and the commencement of formal education, which generally coincides with the start of primary school. Children begin to develop strong relationships with peers and are confronted with being intensely judged for the first time. During middle childhood, school becomes an important part of a child's life, extending their world beyond the family boundaries. Peers start to play a central role, influencing parent-child relationships. Peer acceptance also affects children's self-perception and can have implications for their emotional development in later years (Hoferichter et al., 2021). Entering the world of peers provides many opportunities and can be a positive experience; however, it can also be harmful if the child experiences peer rejection as well as being neglected by adults. Relationships with peers are crucial for children's psychological well-being, reflecting the positive links between peer support and the mental well-being of students, such as joy, a sense of belonging, and the absence of anxiety or boredom. These relationships are important not only for mental health but also for the neurobiological functioning of children's brains (Raufelder et al., 2021). A positive and encouraging school environment can support a child's emotional development, whereas stressful environments and a lack of support can harm it, leading to mental health issues and educational failures (Roeser et al., 2000). Children's experiences at school are shaped not only by interactions with peers, teachers, and staff but also by their perceptions of the school's norms and values, which create a school climate (Hamre & Pianta, 2005). In this chapter on middle childhood, we will focus on several phenomena related to emotional neglect, which, from our perspective, significantly impact the social, emotional, and cognitive development of children

DOI: 10.4324/9781032621203-7

during this period of life. Of course, this catalog is not exhaustive. Analysing these phenomena will help to understand how Social and Emotional Learning (SEL) programmes in schools support the development of key social and emotional skills, which are foundational for mental health and effective functioning in school and social settings.

Understanding peer rejection enables better preparation of intervention strategies and provides support for children experiencing this painful phenomenon. A sense of humour plays an important role in emotional and social development and is also an indicator of mental health. Its development in children often translates into better stress management and stronger relationships with others. The issue of inadequate academic achievement can lead to frustration, low self-esteem, and discouragement, directly affecting children's future educational and vocational opportunities. Lastly, sociocultural challenges and difficulties in regulating tension can drive the development of serious developmental problems and disorders in children. Considering the various areas of functioning in school-aged children allows for a more integrated approach to education and support for children who have experienced emotional neglect from significant adults.

Entering the world of education means immersing oneself in a completely new environment that is full of challenges and changes. Facing new relationships, both with peers and teachers, and adapting to educational requirements, pose tasks that require not only intellectual skills but, above all, the development of emotional competencies (Pan & Zhang, 2023). In the school context, where children interact with a wide spectrum of people, emotional skills are essential for effective adaptation and educational success. The emotional support children receive from teachers and parents is fundamental to their emotional well-being and learning success (Maguire et al., 2016; Sousa et al., 2023). Stable positive relationships with teachers provide children with a safe base from which they can explore and adapt to the school environment (Hamre & Pianta, 2001). Teachers, through active listening, empathy, and appropriate responses to students' emotional needs, can significantly contribute to their social and academic development (Maguire et al., 2016).

Children experiencing emotional neglect often have poor social skills, difficulties in forming or developing friendships (Maguire et al., 2015) and weak emotional regulation skills (Shipman et al., 2005). Studies among children aged 6 to12 years have shown that those who experience neglect exhibit greater peer rejection as they age (Kim & Cicchetti, 2010). Furthermore, Kendall-Tackett and Eckenrode (1996) observed that children aged 11–14 who were neglected had more disciplinary problems and a reduced ability to cope in school.

Emotional neglect and functioning at school

Neglect, including emotional neglect, is associated with the risk of disrupted development in children and deterioration in their overall academic performance

(De Paúl & Arruabarrena, 1995). For example, neglect negatively impacts children's receptive vocabulary (Kantor et al., 2004). Studies have shown that the greater the degree of neglect, the greater the deterioration in vocabulary skills of children aged 6 to 9 years. Similarly, neglect is associated with poorer performance in mathematics, spelling and reading (Kendall-Tackett & Eckenrode, 1996; Reyome, 1993) as well as in tasks involving manual dexterity, auditory attention, visuo-motor integration, flexibility, and complex attention (Nolin & Ethier, 2007). Interestingly, in the study by Nolin and Ethier (2007), emotionally neglected children performed better in tasks requiring problem solving and planning than children who had not experienced neglect. It can be assumed that these children developed compensatory mechanisms that enabled them to respond better to their social expectations. Compensatory strategies may also be activated in other areas such as self-esteem and peer relationships. Finzi et al. (2003), studying Israeli children aged 6–12, found that neglected children more often used compensatory behaviours in social situations, such as acting as the "prankster" or trying to be the "strong guy" in the classroom.

Given the challenges faced by children experiencing emotional neglect, the need for support at the educational level has become evident. While research results indicate significant problems in the academic functioning of these children, a response to these difficulties can be found in the implementation of Social and Emotional Learning (SEL) programmes. SEL is viewed as crucial for children's success in school, especially during the transition from preschool to kindergarten and elementary school (Daunic et al., 2023; Rademacher et al., 2021). Currently, SEL is becoming a priority in modern schools (Tran-Chi et al., 2023) as it plays an important role in students' self-development (Surya et al., 2023). SEL is the process of acquiring key skills that enable understanding and controlling one's emotions, setting and achieving ambitious goals, empathetically perceiving others' positions, building and maintaining healthy relationships, making thoughtful decisions, and effectively managing interactions with others (Duong & Bradshaw, 2017; Elias et al., 1997).

It is also important to note that children exposed to early life stress, which includes violence and neglect, show a reduced volume of the amygdala – a key brain structure involved in emotional and empathetic processes (Hanson et al., 2015).

Recognising and interpreting emotions are key social skills that children develop in elementary education, with the ability to identify emotions improving significantly during this developmental period (Selman, 1981). School-age children become increasingly aware of their own emotional states, and their expressions begin to individualise more. Each child finds their own way to express emotions, requiring high sensitivity and attention from parents, teachers, and other significant adults to resonate and respond appropriately to the emotions experienced by the child. In the school context, the ability to understand emotions directly influences children's behaviour and ability to learn (Maguire et al., 2016). Children who can correctly identify and interpret emotions are more likely to engage in constructive interactions with their peers and teachers. Such emotional competence can contribute to creating a positive classroom atmosphere that supports learning and cooperation (Zins & Elias, 2006). On the other hand, children who struggle to identify and interpret emotions may experience frustration and misunderstanding, leading to externalising behaviours such as aggression, class disruptions, or other forms of lesson disturbance. An inability to understand emotional contexts can result in difficulties adapting to the school environment, which, in turn, impacts the educational process not only for the individual student but also for the entire class (Raver et al., 2007).

Social and emotional learning

In the school environment, Social and Emotional Learning (SEL) comprises two sets of coordinated educational strategies aimed at enhancing school achievement and supporting student development (CASEL, 2022; McCormick et al., 2015). First, enhancing school achievement, where SEL strategies are designed to help students better manage school demands, including self-awareness – recognising; self-management – being; social awareness – showing; relationship skills; and responsible decision-making and problem solving. Children can achieve better academic outcomes by improving their competency in social and emotional skills (Durlak et al., 2011). Second, in supporting student development, beyond just academic achievement, SEL also focuses on students' emotional and social development. SEL programmes teach students how to recognise and manage their emotions, build healthy relationships, make responsible decisions, and empathise. These skills are essential for effective functioning in school, at home, and in society.

School climate refers to the overall quality and atmosphere of school life, shaped by the experiences of its members, and it forms an important social context for children and youth. It encompasses norms, values, relationships, teaching and learning practices, and organisational structures (Sousa et al., 2023), support for students, support for teachers, and opportunities for autonomy (Jia et al., 2009; Zhao et al., 2023). A positive and balanced school climate encourages youth development and prepares them for success in society. It also promotes a sense of safety and engagement, and encourages collaboration among students, families, and teachers to achieve a shared vision of the school (Wang et al., 2013). While individual experiences influence school climate, it is ultimately a group phenomenon that encompasses various aspects of school life and organisational patterns (Cohen et al., 2009). According to Bronfenbrenner's psychosocial ecological theory, which relates to the influence of different environmental levels on human development, individual factors such as sensitivity to rejection (which may be a result of emotional neglect) and the school climate can together affect the emergence of aggression among students (Hong & Espelage, 2012).

Due to still-developing conceptual thinking (which requires concrete actions), school-age children learn better through active participation rather than passive listening. Therefore, "educational" discussions about relationships are insufficient, and children need to engage in real relationships. The role of an adult is to gently oversee this process and provide support when necessary. Knowledge is also more easily absorbed when embedded in real-life contexts, allowing children to see practical applications of what they are learning. Adults become essential guides in reality, bearing the responsibility of creating conditions for learning that cater to a child's personal curiosity and preferences. How parents handle their "adult" responsibilities, whether they find satisfaction in them, will influence what is modelled for their children.

Challenges to emotion regulation

While the school environment is becoming increasingly important for a child's daily life, the home setting and family relationships continue to play a significant role in the development and functioning of school-age children. Parents find it increasingly difficult to read their children's emotional states as children develop skills to hide their feelings and may even deny them. However, high parental sensitivity and previously established good relationships with the child enable the detection of problematic situations such as bullying, peer relationship difficulties, violence, or inadequate emotional regulation. Poor management of emotional stress can lead to many negative consequences, among which we will focus on two serious phenomena that have escalated in the 21st century: substance use and overeating.

Another very serious problem related to improper emotional regulation and disturbed parent-child relationships is children's use of psychoactive substances. In children with depressive and anxiety issues, which often result from emotional neglect, there is an increased risk of experimenting with psychoactive substances (Thomasius et al., 2022). We discuss substance abuse further in the next chapter.

In school-age children, the increasing problem of obesity (Abarca-Gómez et al., 2017), including severe obesity (Spinelli et al., 2019), is concerning because at this age, parents are primarily responsible for preparing meals and shaping and overseeing their children's eating habits. Food serves not only a nutritional function but is also a significant means of regulating emotions (Macht, 2008). Children may discover on their own that eating (or consuming specific types of food such as carbohydrates) can be calming. Furthermore, Kininmonth et al. (2021) in their review showed that the tendency towards obesity appears more pronounced in children with greater access to high-calorie foods and screens in their bedrooms. This observation aligns with the assumption that children prefer quick ways of soothing their emotions. However, parents often participate in this process, offering sweets to manage their child's stress. The quick-calming effect combined with minimal effort fits well within a right-thumb mentality, where quick and easy solutions are prioritised and reinforced. While it is difficult to expect deep reflection and high emotional self-regulation skills from school-aged children, especially younger ones, such expectations can be placed on their parents. However, in the hustle of life, and with easy access to junk food and sweets, parents may opt for immediate and rewarding solutions. Often, they blame the child for long-term effects such as weight gain, demanding a corrective plan from them. However, the example set by the parents themselves is crucial. Research on childhood obesity has shown various and sometimes contradictory results, suggesting that the development of obesity in children is rather a transactional process involving biological, interpersonal, and family factors (Clément & Tereno, 2023).

The issue of childhood obesity and parental support in the process of regaining a healthy weight is crucial because obesity is a risk factor for many metabolic diseases, contributes to affective disorders, limits a child's ability to engage in physically demanding activities, and affects the child's body image and self-esteem. Neglecting the problem of obesity in childhood can have very negative consequences for the child's future functioning. Identifying the causes of excessive weight and implementing interventions involving the entire family system can help mitigate these consequences. Again, attention to the child, empathy and modelling healthy emotional habits, including coping with emotional distress, by parents, are critical in this process.

One of the healthier strategies for regulating emotions and building social relationships that develops during middle childhood is a sense of humour. Humour helps establish and maintain social relationships, and sharing laughter can foster bonds and a sense of belonging. McGhee (2010) emphasises that developing a sense of humour in children is crucial for their ability to cope with stress, adapt to new situations, and build emotional resilience. Humour can also serve as a tool for exploring one's identity and expressing creativity (Cann & Collette, 2014). Emotional neglect can lead to maladaptive styles of humour. Research by Kazarian et al. (2010) has shown that those who remember being accepted by their mothers and fathers more often use adaptive humour styles that reinforce both themselves and others. On the other hand, those who remember being rejected by their parents tend to use maladaptive humour styles that promote devaluation of oneself and or other people.

Starting in preschool, the first signs of children's ability to understand and express humour can be identified (Klein & Kuiper, 2006). However, it is during middle childhood, between the ages of 6 and 12, that humour begins to play a significantly more important role, becoming a tool for effective functioning within the community and a means of building relationships with peers (Bergen, 1998). In middle childhood, children learn to function in larger social groups, and their interaction skills are tested. Humour can be a valuable asset in this context. Children who effectively use humour often enjoy greater acceptance among their peers, which translates to better social relationships (Martin et al., 2003). They may find it easier to make new friends, perceive themselves as more socially attractive, and often play a central role in their group. On the other hand, a lack of humour skills or its inappropriate use can lead to difficulties in peer relationships (Burger, 2022). Children who cannot engage in humorous exchanges with others or whose attempts at humour are misunderstood or inappropriate may face rejection, which can consequently lead to social isolation, lower self-esteem, and emotional problems.

Peer relationships

Rejection is another challenge faced by children aged 6 to12 years. Upon starting elementary school, peer relationships become increasingly important for children seeking close and safe bonds with their peers (Feng & Zhou, 2023). However, not everyone has had positive experiences with these relationships. Peer rejection occurs when a person is ignored or rejected by a group, and this phenomenon is often associated with ostracism (Williams, 2007). Some researchers, observing the effects of rejection on children's personality development, describe it in terms of personality traits (see Dodge et al., 2003).

Children who struggle to establish positive relationships with peers during early and middle childhood are more likely to perform poorly in school, skip classes, and drop out of school prematurely than children who do not have peer-related issues during these developmental stages (DeRosier et al., 1994; Kupersmidt & Coie, 1990; Woodward & Fergusson, 2000). These children are more frequently observed to have behavioural, adaptive, and mental health disorders (Di Giunta et al., 2018). Oncioiu et al. (2020) in their longitudinal study analysed the development of peer victimisation from ages 6 to 17 years and its relationship with early childhood behaviour and family traits. The researchers identified four different patterns of peer victimisation during compulsory education: low, moderate-emerging, childhood-limited, and high-chronic. Some children experienced continual victimisation in elementary school, which was linked to externalising behaviours and family weaknesses in early childhood.

Healthy functioning within the family can serve as a buffer against experiences of rejection. On the other hand, parents can take appropriate interventions in cases of peer violence towards their children and help them cope with the consequences of unpleasant experiences. These actions require parental engagement and good communication with children. Parents can also manipulate the conditions of their child's environment to make them safer, for example by avoiding difficult situations for the child. This solution may be easier for parents. However, especially for younger children, parents play a role in ensuring opportunities for spontaneous relationships with peers. However, increasingly, in the spirit of caring for a child's welfare, excessive parental control over interactions with other children is observed. Parents choose the school (the best for the child from an adult's perspective), often far from home, and provide organised after-school activities. While this fosters the development of certain skills in the child, it also prevents them from practising the nuances of interpersonal skirmishes and games. It is in peer relationships, especially friendships, that children learn to resolve conflicts and endure the discomfort associated with differing opinions (Boyd & Bee, 2013).

Functioning in a group has another important function for school-aged children. Observing others and comparing oneself with them is an important mechanism for building one's own global self-esteem. This process begins to develop rapidly from the age of 7 years. Self-esteem largely results from the discrepancy between how the child would like to be (ideal self) and how they perceive themselves in reality (real self). Therefore, the influence of environmental factors is crucial. For the assessment of the real self, how the child is perceived by their close peers and what is reflected back to them will be significant. Children who receive signals that they are liked as they are will have a higher sense of self-worth. Meanwhile, the ideal self is closely related to desired models in a particular social group. Here, it is crucial to compare oneself with others, including ideal models. In the age of the Internet, every child has the opportunity to compare not only with their immediate circle of friends (see Dunbar's number, Chapter 3), but practically with the whole world. This means that there will always be many people who are better at something, more capable, better looking, etc. Whatever a child does, there will always be someone who can do it more, better, and faster. On the other hand, commenting on content published on social media can work in both ways: it allows the creation of a support network, but also exposes the child to unpleasant information and hate, which is facilitated by anonymity on the Internet.

Parental burnout

Overseeing the above processes falls on the parents. Contemporary society is characterised by a fast-paced life, high professional expectations, and increased educational pressure. In this context, parents often struggle with the challenges brought by engagement in professional life and simultaneously meeting the emotional needs of their children. Modern educational systems (in most countries) are criticised for focusing excessively on outcomes and academic metrics at the expense of areas such as creativity, empathy, and abilities. Psychologists and educators clearly indicate that children need a significant amount of time spent with their parents, and emotional support, for healthy development. A lack of such support can lead to behavioural and emotional problems in children, as demonstrated in previous chapters of this book. Today, it is difficult for parents and caregivers to find a balance between professional demands and family life. Work hours are extending (which is not always due to economic situations or the organisation of a particular job position), numerous responsibilities related to managing children's education add up, and parents try to meet their own needs, pumped up by a right-thumb mentality (see Chapter 2).

When the burden associated with childcare exceeds parents' ability to cope with these stresses, there is a risk of parental burnout (Mikolajczak et al., 2019). This state, like professional burnout, is characterised by three main features. First, is the exhaustion associated with the parent's role. Parents feel tired and drained by their responsibilities, which result from continuous care for a child or children. Exhaustion can manifest both physically and emotionally. The second feature of parental burnout is emotional distancing from children. Parents may feel emotionally detached from their children, experience less engagement in their lives, or have difficulty in showing affection. The third characteristic of parental burnout is a diminished sense of accomplishment as a parent. Parents may feel that they are not meeting their expectations of themselves as caregivers, which can lead to feelings of failure and low self-esteem (Roskam et al., 2018).

Studies show that parents suffering from burnout are more likely to abuse and neglect their children, exposing them to harmful effects in both the short and long term (Griffith, 2022). It should also be mentioned that parental burnout is different to professional burnout, but a small correlation between these phenomena has been demonstrated (Mikolajczak et al., 2019; Roskam et al., 2018; Van Bakel et al., 2022).

Interestingly, parental burnout can also be a result of medicalisation, in which physiological exhaustion from an overload of responsibilities and challenges is more easily referred to in "medical" terms, thereby obtaining permission to publicly express the difficult emotions resulting from parenting (see Chapter 2).

Education anxiety

Education Anxiety (Chen & Xiao, 2014) is another phenomenon that can influence parents' emotional neglect of their children. Educational anxiety is a state of anxiety experienced by parents (a phenomenon particularly noticeable in some Asian countries) owing to high expectations, uncertainty of educational outcomes, and fear of their children's failure. This anxiety can manifest at various stages of a child's development and is often influenced by social pressure to achieve excellent academic results. When children enter middle school, parents may experience increased anxiety due to the rapid physical and mental development of the child and reduced communication between parents and children (Wu et al., 2022). Wu et al. (2022) found a positive correlation between parental education-related anxiety and the level of parental burnout. This means that the greater the anxiety about the child's education, the higher the level of burnout among parents. Considering the findings of the above studies and that emotional abuse can have negative consequences on students' educational achievements, considering that emotional well-being is significantly associated with the risk of underachievement (Hoffmann, 2020), this could further reinforce Education Anxiety, however, this is a hypothesis that would need to be confirmed by research studies. Underachievement is a profound discrepancy between students' school performance and indicators of their actual capabilities such as intelligence, creativity, curiosity about the world, and a keen sense of observation (Arega, 2023).

Expectations in the child-parent relationship

In summary, during school age, parents bear many responsibilities, some of which are conditioned not so much by the needs of the child (e.g., patiently and delicately adjusting support and reinforcing the child's self-esteem), but by socio-cultural influences (e.g., ensuring the child's educational success). These various tasks can be in opposition and even create a vicious cycle, worsening the functioning of both the child and parent, as is illustrated in Figure 7.1.

The need for compensatory actions (e.g., for low self-esteem), such as ensuring a good start in life for the child, being a good parent, ensuring the child's safety, being in touch with the child, and providing the child with high material status, can lead to excessive involvement in various activities. This results in a permanent lack of time, depletion of resources, deprivation of personal needs, and consequently, an increase in negative affect that must be discharged through compensatory strategies. Meanwhile, lack of time and decreasing effectiveness lead to parents not achieving their intended outcomes, which contributes to worsening self-esteem and self-image as a parent.

An almost identical process can occur on the child's side. To meet the demands imposed by parents and the environment, children may face their own inadequacies (insufficient resources and lack of time), leading to disappointment and low self-esteem. Similarly, by not receiving what they need from the parent, the child may feel let down and perceive themselves as unworthy of attention. To compensate for low self-esteem, the child may undertake efforts that exceed their capabilities and consume resources, leading to deprivation of needs and escalation of problems that they experience.

On both sides of the parent-child dyad, self-esteem deteriorates, frustration builds, and a sense of misunderstanding grows. To break these mutually

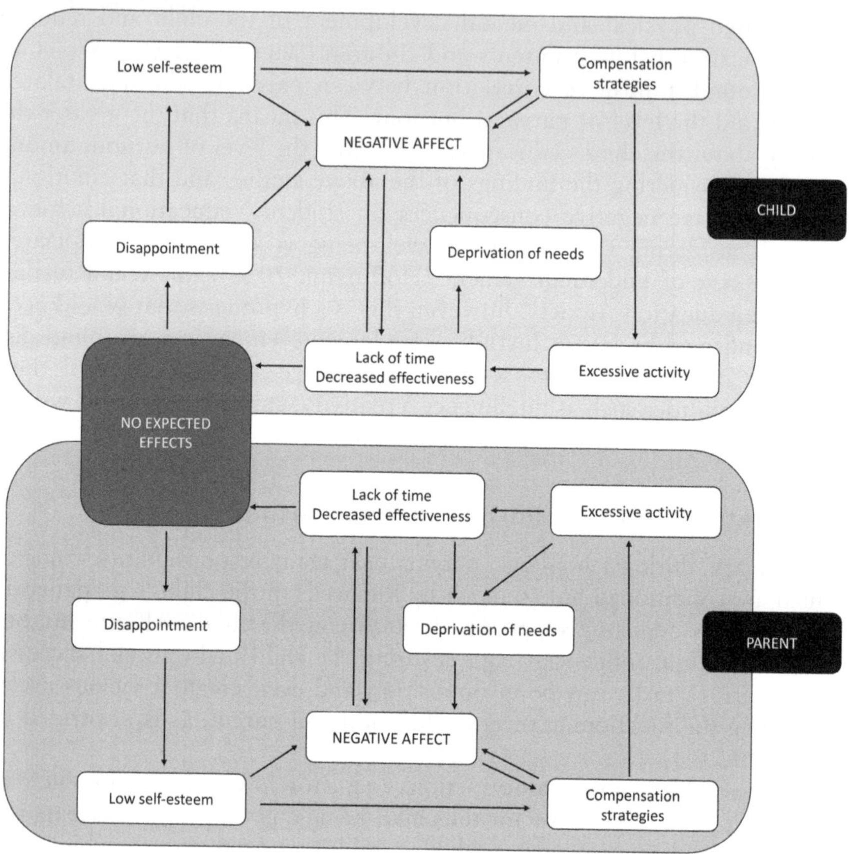

Figure 7.1 The vicious circle of not meeting expectations in the child-parent relationship.

reinforcing vicious cycles in the parent-child dyad, communication becomes fundamental, particularly regarding the needs and emotions experienced, taking into account both one's own and the other's perspective. Such discussions are more effective in resolving problems and satisfying needs, and consequently, these effects extend beyond the parent-child dyad and lead to a general improvement in social skills and competencies (Fenning et al., 2011).

Chapter 8

Adolescence

Find your own place and recognise yourself

Challenges and potential issues in the period of adolescences

Key tasks in adolescence are the development of personal autonomy, identity, interpersonal skills and self-worth. Separating from the familial generational system involves verifying and identifying one's values, building and learning about romantic and friendship relationships, cultivating curiosity about the world and creating openness to diversity and differences. This requires parental trust, safely loosening the parent-child bond and allowing adolescents to draw from the experiences of others, especially emotional ones. During this developmental period, young individuals begin to utilise their emotions independently to establish their own system of relationships and support. For the first time, they also have the resources to independently manage their boundaries and recognise those of others. When young people experience emotional neglect, it can lead to several negative consequences such as an increased likelihood of antisocial behaviours or juvenile delinquency (Tornberry et al., 2001). In addition, emotional neglect increases the risk of mental health disorders (Jessar et al., 2017), such as affective disorders (Epkins & Heckler, 2011), eating disorders (Amianto et al., 2018; Caslini et al., 2016; Dawson et al., 2022; Mills et al., 2015.), dissociative disorders (Dorahy et al., 2016), personality disorders (Wildschut et al., 2020), addiction (Nazlıgül et al., 2023), as well as procrastination (Ma & Song, 2023) and becoming a school dropout (Choe, 2021). Emotional neglect during childhood can double the risk of depression in adulthood and is a primary factor in the increased rate of adult suicide (Angelakis et al., 2020; Damian et al., 2021).

Building autonomy and self

Adolescence is a crucial time for the formation of identity, marked by a struggle between identity confusion and integration (Erikson, 1968). While the quest for autonomy comes to the forefront, emotional support from adults

DOI: 10.4324/9781032621203-8

is essential during this period for healthy psychological and emotional development of adolescents. Identity development in adolescence is a complex process in which young people explore various aspects of themselves to build a coherent sense of identity (Marcia, 1966). Identity involves dynamic processes that shape the sense of one's "self" in interactions between the adolescent and broader structures such as social systems.

Identity is defined as the awareness of being an integrated, unique individual who finds a balance between personal and social needs, possesses an understanding of their own life history, and has a framework that guides their behaviour (Abels, 2010). As a social being, a person's identity is born through communication with the environment and requires conflict resolution throughout development (Erikson, 1968). It is a process of continual confrontations and verification of one's previous vision of themselves and the world, and often a difficult process arousing many negative emotions. Adolescents predominantly experience negative affect over positive emotions (Abitante et al., 2022) and when adolescents' experiences reach the level of trauma, there can be disturbances in their identity development (Lawson & Quinn, 2013). Adolescents who struggle with conflicts and have been exposed to emotional neglect are at risk of developing identity diffusion, which is the opposite of an integrated identity (Igarashi et al., 2009; Penner et al., 2019).

Identity diffusion is associated with a persistent sense of discomfort arising from ambivalence, a lack of meaning, and prevailing regret or sadness. To alleviate this discomfort, adolescents may seek answers to questions about the purpose of their existence and identity from external sources. As a result, they are highly susceptible to radical influences. They may engage in religious groups, activist movements or extremist groups (see Isenhardt et al., 2021). This aligns with the Uncertainty-Identity Theory (Hogg, 2013), which suggests that individuals uncertain of their identity are more likely to identify with groups that provide a clearly defined identity, beliefs and behavioural patterns. In such cases, young people stop developing an autonomous self in favour of an identity merged with the group's agenda, where they find acceptance. However, this acceptance is conditional: "you belong with us as long as you respect our rules". It is worth noting that adolescents who have experienced healthy conditions in their family home, whose parents were involved and developed a healthy bond with their children, were less susceptible to the influence of peer groups (Xie et al., 2023).

Moreover, identity confusion is a risk factor for engaging in self-destructive behaviours, primarily non-suicidal self-injury (Breen et al., 2013; Claes et al., 2014; Hou et al. 2023). In families where there is space for non-judgemental conversations and openness to emotional exchange, it is much easier to resolve adolescents' problems or at least help them cope with tension. In poorly functioning families where emotional neglect is more common, the risk of non-suicidal self-injury increases (Cassels et al., 2018; Nemati et al., 2020)

Self-esteem, self-confidence and a sense of self-efficacy are crucial traits that determine how young people perceive their futures. Feelings of hopelessness and pessimism about the future, along with reduced self-worth, often result from emotional neglect and developmental trauma (Domke et al., 2023; Howe, 2005). Emotional neglect and excessive criticism also give rise to what is known as the "inner critic", which sustains negative beliefs about oneself and the world (Gilbert, 2000). These phenomena can consequently lead to disturbances in the process of building close relationships, including intimate ones.

Need for uniqueness

The need for uniqueness, described 50 years ago as an individual's desire to stand out and be distinct from others (Snyder & Fromkin, 1977), remains a key motive in the process of identity formation (Vignoles et al., 2011). Uniqueness on the one hand fits into contemporary manifestations of right-thumb mentality (see Chapter 2), yet on the other, it may clash with the lack of approval in more conservative religious environments (e.g., "one must be modest") or collectivist cultures (Burns & Brady, 1992; Vignoles et al., 2000).

Uniqueness can be an aim in itself, but it can also serve as a means of achieving other goals and values. Individualism, which is dominating and increasingly occurring, even in collectivist cultures (Cai et al., 2018), enhances the need for self-expression. A right-thumb mentality pushes this need even further, therefore, finding clear, preferably measurable indicators of this uniqueness becomes necessary. Popularity can serve such a role (Santor et al., 2000; Wright, 2018). The development of new technologies has enabled an increase in the reach of one's popularity, which explains why young people are so engaged in social media. However, these same media expose an individual to the activities and uniqueness of people from all over the world. Suddenly, it turns out that a unique idea has long been in place elsewhere and that others are doing something similar. Attempts to replicate unique ideas or activities lead to maximum reproduction. Authentic uniqueness is reduced to common repeatability. The need to stand out above this level necessitates doing something extreme, shocking, or quirky, often no longer a reflection of an adolescent's authentic identity but rather a creation aimed at being noticed and recognised by important people in the adolescent's life. Adolescents who have experienced emotional neglect and who have not been "seen" by their close ones may be particularly susceptible to this.

It is also worth noting that the increasing difficulty of standing out among others and the necessity for artificial self-creation can discourage efforts in this area. If success in uniqueness is not achievable, it makes no sense to invest resources in it. This can lead to a risk of adolescents withdrawing into inactivity, in line with Seligman's (1974) concept of learned helplessness.

A lack of achievement and a decrease in activity are significant factors that contribute to depression (López-López et al., 2021). Thus, a situation arises in which two tendencies clash: the need for uniqueness and the need to withdraw from an unrealistic rat race. Compensatory strategies and depression are intertwined. Zhang & Zhang (2023) have demonstrated that depression acts as a mediator between the need for uniqueness and non-suicidal self-injury.

Gender identity

One area of personal identity that is especially crucial during adolescence is gender identity. Physical maturation and the development of sexual characteristics associated with biologically determined gender present a challenge for every teenager. Physical and hormonal changes in the body can significantly alter an adolescent's functioning. It is difficult to accept and adapt to these changes. There are increasingly highlighted issues young people face regarding gender identity since, in recent years, there has been a significant increase in the number of terms used to describe gender identities, leading to the discovery of more specific types and subtypes (Watson et al., 2020).

Adolescence is a time of self-discovery and the process of exploring one's gender identity may proceed at a different pace for everyone. This can be problematic when young people are pushed into specific gender roles by external environments based solely on their biological sex. Disregarding teenagers' feelings, minimising their opinions, and denying their explorations are examples of neglect by adults, who during this phase of life should play a supportive but not dominating role. Attentiveness, sensitivity, and openness to conversation among adults are crucial.

Empirical data suggest that individuals who identify with less "standard" gender identities are at a higher risk of mental health disorders and discrimination (O'Leary et al., 2024; Veale et al., 2017). A study by Borgogna et al. (2019) found that individuals identified as queer and pansexual experience higher rates of depression and anxiety than those who identify as gay or lesbian. Among non-binary youths, there is a higher rate of self-harm and increased emotional distress (Veale et al., 2017). These findings underscore the critical importance of and need for healthy relationships with close associates who can provide young people with a platform for safely exploring their gender identity and for having open discussions about their experiences and views in this area.

Emotionality in adolescence

Teenagers' emotions are highly turbulent. Their capacity for emotional self-regulation is very unstable and susceptible to external environmental influences as well as internal ones, such as hormonal and emotional changes.

To explain this instability, a neurobiological model based on the competition between neuronal systems processing emotional and cognitive control systems is often used (Casey et al., 2019; Schulman et al., 2016). Meanwhile, the imbalance model (Casey et al., 2019; Luna & Wright, 2016) suggests that the neuronal circuits that regulate emotions mature and fine-tune at different times. Subcortical circuits, including the amygdala, mature earlier than cortico-subcortical and cortical circuits do. This explains why adolescents often display impulsive behaviour in situations of strong emotional arousal (Sommerville et al., 2011). The neuronal circuits involved in emotional self-regulation typically reach maturity after 21 years of age (Casey et al., 2019).

Alongside neuronal maturity for emotional self-regulation, the cognitive belief that emotions can be controlled is also crucial. This is part of the process of forming emotional schemas (Leahy, 2015), which are beliefs about emotions (their significance, controllability, duration, etc.), the feelings associated with these beliefs, and corresponding behaviours. In the emotional schema model, emotions are objects for thinking, not merely the results of thinking, as posited in cognitive models of emotion (e.g., Beck, 2011).

Emotional schemas are formed through learning, in which instruction from older and more experienced individuals is paramount. Emotions are always anchored in context. Emotion itself is merely a signal; it is the cognitive processing of the context that reveals the true need and significance of this signal. Emotional schemas develop throughout a person's life, and earlier developmental phases are crucial in this process (Di Giunta et al., 2022). However, adolescence introduces new phenomena and challenges in parent-child relationships that can significantly influence these schemas. Parental desires to protect their child from the dangers of independent living, or to limit the child's autonomy in favour of obedience, can further reinforce the formation of maladaptive emotional schemas. These schemas often relate to undesired and problematic beliefs about emotionality, such as "emotions are unbearable, they will never end", "I can't control my anger", or "if I feel fear, it means I am weak". Meanwhile, the role of an emotionally engaged parent would be to support the child in building and, especially during adolescence, reassessing emotional schemas that include solutions, such as "sadness signifies something important, I can explore it and thus better appreciate my life". Although contemporary culture often discusses emotions, the favoured approach is still to control emotions in the sense of not displaying them in difficult situations. Emotion regulation in adolescents occurs not only through interactions with adults but also within peer groups, intertwining emotional experiences and relationships with other young people.

Adolescent relationships

Adolescent relationships are a blend of family interactions, friendships, intimate connections, and increasingly, virtual relationships. The use of social networks by teenagers is expanding, encompassing more of their daily activities. Over half of the global population uses social media (Dam et al., 2023), and this mode of maintaining contacts has become the norm for teenagers. Many teenagers are engaging in building their reach and increasing the number of followers. While this allows some to earn income or fame, for many others it results in activities that ultimately isolate them from everyday functional opportunities. The amount and quality of time spent online are linked to the risk of depressive and anxiety symptoms, sleep deterioration, and media addiction (Dam et al., 2023; Demircioğlu & Göncü-Köse, 2023; Karim et al., 2020; Twenge & Campbell, 2018).

The postmodern right-thumb mentality demands achieving as many goals as possible in the shortest time, requiring people to remain updated. Social media satisfies this need, but also intensifies a phenomenon known as the fear of missing out (FOMO) (Alutaybi et al., 2020). Using social media helps meet important psychological needs, such as staying connected to others (Fabris et al., 2020). Fabris et al. (2020) also show that spending more time online can be associated with the fear of receiving negative comments or not getting enough likes. Moreover, studies have indicated that more problematic use of social media and the Internet is found in individuals with insecure attachment styles (Gori et al., 2023), which is directly linked to emotional neglect.

As mentioned, social media can help establish and maintain contacts with other important people; however, the phenomenon of "phubbing" is concurrently evolving (Xie et al., 2023). Phubbing involves neglecting the person one is physically with in favour of engaging with a smartphone. Studies have shown that such behaviour negatively impacts relationship quality and intimacy of interactions, and increases conflicts (Xie et al., 2023; Vanden Abeele et al., 2019; Beukeboom & Pollmann, 2021).

It appears that contemporary threats to adolescent relationships primarily involve a lack of time to build deeper relationships, fostering superficial acquaintances (quantity over quality of relationships), and difficulty tolerating the emotional discomfort that naturally arises in close relationships. Virtual relationships are increasingly less facilitative of emotional development for adolescents and parents, who themselves succumb to virtual realities and phubbing, increasingly lacking space to accompany and model face-to-face relationships for their teenagers (Xie et al., 2023).

Friendship

Sullivan (1953), in his theory of interpersonal relations, argued that interactions between people are foundational for personality development. Sullivan emphasised that the quality of these interactions can have a lasting impact on an individual's mental well-being. Friendships during adolescence can offer a unique space for exploring one's identity and emotions and developing interpersonal skills, which is especially crucial for those who have experienced emotional neglect in childhood. As noted by Zhao et al. (2021), in the face of emotional neglect, girls are more likely than boys to seek emotional support in friendships with their peers. The quality of friendships plays a significant role (Berndt, 2004; Dong et al., 2023) and can mitigate the link between experiencing emotional neglect in childhood and a negative self-image. It appears that the negative impact of experienced neglect on self-perception is stronger among youth who have lower-quality friendship relations. In other words, if an adolescent has friends who do not provide support, understanding, and acceptance, negative beliefs about oneself, stemming from emotional neglect in childhood, are more likely to intensify (Li et al., 2023). High-quality friendships, characterised by reciprocity, trust, and support, can be particularly helpful in building self-compassion among adolescents who have experienced emotional neglect (Dong et al., 2023). Moreover, as the quality of friendships improves, the impact that emotional neglect from childhood has on deepening depression decreases.

As relationships among teenagers deepen, the topics of their conversations change, often including difficult subjects. Adolescents at this developmental stage may struggle to balance compassion by distancing themselves from the suffering of others. Often, teenagers try to "rescue" their interlocutors (though they lack the resources to do so) or avoid difficult topics. Empathising can become too burdensome, and by avoiding difficult conversations, teenagers may consequently experience deterioration in relationships (Eisenberg, 2000).

Romantic relationships

During adolescence, romantic relationships are usually not long lasting and are highly susceptible to external factors. However, these relationships begin to play a crucial role in young people's emotional and social development. Behavioural patterns and attitudes learned from one's family have a significant impact on shaping these relationships. Insecure attachment styles can manifest as difficulties in trusting a partner, avoiding closeness, excessive emotional dependency, or difficulties in emotional communication. These challenges can lead to conflicts, reduced satisfaction within relationships, and problems in maintaining stable and fulfilling romantic relationships (Collins et al., 2009). Individuals who have experienced mistreatment in childhood, including emotional neglect, tend to form less stable relationships (Mullen et al., 1996; Sun et al., 2021), which are more dysfunctional (DiLillo et al., 2009), conflict-prone (Briere & Rickards, 2007; Handley et al., 2021), characterised by limited trust (Sun et al., 2021), emotional dysregulation (Bradbury & Shaffer, 2012), and low relationship quality (Cao et al., 2022; Reyome, 2010).

Romantic relationships also involve adolescents' engagement in sexual relationships. Peer group pressures and familial patterns (Tomé et al., 2012) can lead to engaging in sexual activity before an adolescent is ready. In families in which children have developed an insecure attachment style, there is a much higher occurrence of premature sexual initiation. Relationships are often with casual partners and are frequently accompanied by experiences of violence (Yarkovsky et al., 2014).

One of the more serious consequences of adolescent sexual activity is teenage pregnancy, a significant issue primarily in developing countries, but also present in developed ones (WHO, 2024). A major factor contributing to this issue is the coercion of girls into sexual activity, either through mechanisms of sexual violence or for sociocultural reasons. For instance, it is estimated that in 2021, around 120 million girls under the age of 20 were victims of sexual violence by someone other than a partner, and approximately 650 million girls entered into marriages, although child marriage is considered a violation of human rights. Often, girls who marry early have no say in choosing their partner, their autonomy is significantly restricted, and they usually have no control over the decision to become pregnant because of limited access to contraceptives.

The issue of lack of access to contraceptives is not only a problem in developing countries. Globally, teenagers face challenges in this area, and worse, even when they have access, they often do not know how to use contraception properly. The age of sexual initiation among adolescents is decreasing, but their readiness to form mature and responsible relationships remains limited (Osorio et al., 2017; Young et al., 2018). Many teenagers do not know how to protect themselves against pregnancy or sexually transmitted diseases. There is a widespread lack of formal and informal education (Silva et al., 2022; Vieira Martins et al., 2023). In this case, support, both instrumental and emotional, from parents, and perhaps even more importantly from teachers, educators, and medical staff, is crucial in mitigating the negative consequences that teenagers may face in the realm of sexual activity. A good relationship between adolescents and their parents and close adults appears to be key to safeguarding teenagers (Williams, 2003).

Loneliness

Loneliness refers to the subjective feeling of being alone or isolated, regardless of the actual number or quality of social connections a teenager may have (McWhirter, 1990). This represents a discrepancy between desired and actual levels of social interaction (Majorano et al., 2015). Although loneliness can be chosen and viewed positively as an opportunity for self-reflection or rest, it is typically negatively experienced and can lead to a range of negative health and emotional outcomes (Marcoen et al., 1987). Majorano et al. (2015) note that the motivation for loneliness can have both positive and negative consequences, depending on whether it is autonomous (stemming from internal motivation and needs) or controlled (caused by external factors) and potentially prompted by emotional neglect. Musetti et al. (2021) demonstrated that adolescents who experienced emotional neglect in childhood tended to feel more isolation and exclusion by their parents during adolescence. Their research also showed that teenagers with a history of emotional neglect might develop various strategies for regulating boundaries between themselves and others, which can both intensify and compensate for their feelings of loneliness. Wang and Zhao (2023) found that emotional neglect is more strongly associated with adolescent loneliness than emotional abuse.

Turkle (2011) argued that, while modern technologies are designed to facilitate human contact, they often lead to shallow interactions that do not satisfy deep emotional needs. In the era of social media, people may feel "Alone Together", surrounded by virtual "friends" yet devoid of authentic, meaningful relationships. Adolescents growing in a world dominated by digital media are particularly vulnerable to the negative effects of isolation and loneliness. Orben et al. (2020) emphasise that reducing face-to-face social interactions in favour of digital ones can lead to feelings of isolation and loneliness. Thus, loneliness in the crowd resulting from digital isolation can contribute to an increase in mental health issues, underscoring the need to develop social skills and build deeper personal relationships.

Psychoactive substance abuse

Numerous emotional burdens, school obligations, sociocultural pressures to meet expectations, unsatisfactory relationships, and consumerism, all make the adolescent period particularly painful for modern teenagers. The absence of close emotional relationships, which could buffer experienced difficulties, leads youths to seek other ways to release tension. One of the simplest methods is turning to psychoactive substances. Many teenagers have their first contact with psychoactive substances between the ages of 13 and 15 years (Thomasius et al., 2022).

The opioid addiction pandemic is a contemporary problem that is increasingly affecting adolescents (Gaur et al., 2020; Lyons et al., 2019; Wilson et al., 2020). Opioids also play a crucial role in pain relief. As mentioned in Chapter 3, pain can be induced by the activation of brain structures, including the anterior cingulate cortex (dACC), responsible for processing social stimuli. Experiences such as injustice, relational loss, or exclusion can evoke feelings of physical pain, which may motivate attempts to take pain-relieving drugs. These social experiences are common in teenagers' lives.

Considering that adolescents may use psychoactive substances to regulate emotions, this again highlights the importance of developing healthy self-regulation methods that children should acquire in the earlier stages of their development. The use of psychoactive substances by children and adolescents is particularly problematic. The risks associated with addiction, deterioration of physical and mental health, relationship disorders, and impairment in the ability to develop a healthy autonomous self are evident (Henden, 2023). Adolescents are at a very high risk of addiction (chemical and behavioural), partly due to the development of the reward system involved in addiction processes. The reward system consists of two parts: the reactive system (bottom-up, including subcortical circuits such as the ventral tegmental area and amygdala), the reflective system (top-down, involving the prefrontal cortex), and meeting in the nucleus accumbens (Swartz et al., 2020). The reactive reward system does not include neuronal circuits involved in processing and analysing information, and does not rely on thinking processes. Activation of this system by a psychoactive substance acts as a switch that quickly triggers a reward in the nucleus accumbens. The reflective system can inhibit responses in the nucleus accumbens and, if it deems the intake of a psychoactive substance as dangerous or unprofitable, postpone or completely stop the desire to consume the substance. While the reactive system matures very quickly, the reflective system, which involves cortical structures, matures slower and only achieves operational efficiency in adulthood.

Emotional invalidation

Parents' reactions to children's emotional expressions are important for emotion socialisation (Bennett et al., 2019), as discussed in Chapter 1. Emotional invalidation is a process in which a teenager's expressed emotions are ignored, rejected, downplayed or criticised by another person. This can occur in a variety of contexts such as family, romantic relationships, and friendships. Emotional invalidation can take many forms, including: denying another person's emotional experience, such as saying "you shouldn't feel that way" or "it's not a big deal"; minimising the importance of emotions, such as "don't worry about it so much" or "you're overdramatizing it"; criticising the expression of emotions, such as "only weak people cry" or "don't be so sensitive"; and ignoring or avoiding talking about emotions, such as changing the topic when someone expresses their feelings. Elzy (2013, p. vi) points out that "emotional invalidation is a construct closely related to childhood maltreatment, which has been linked theoretically and empirically to the development of psychopathology". Research by Lambie and Lindberg (2016) indicates that children's ability to focus on their own emotional states–that is, their emotional awareness–may be shaped by the way mothers confirm or deny their child's emotions. Additionally, emotional invalidation may increase the risk of developing eating disorders by negatively affecting body image and self-esteem (Mountford et al., 2007).

Jin et al. (2023) study showed that the experience of emotional neglect in childhood can have a long-term impact on the processing of facial emotions in young adults. They found that people with childhood emotional neglect experience identified emotions in faces more slowly than those in the control group. These results suggest that emotional neglect leads to a delay in facial emotional processing in young adults, which may be related to insufficient, inaccessible, and limited patterns of emotional interactions between parents and children.

In summary the developmental task of adolescence is to develop one's autonomy. Separating from the generational (or nuclear) family system requires verifying and identifying one's values, building and learning romantic and friendly relationships, arousing curiosity about the world and openness to otherness, differences and diversity. What is necessary here is the parent's trust, safely loosening the parent-child bond and the opportunity to draw from other people's experiences – especially the emotional ones. When young people experience neglect, there are many negative consequences, such as an increased likelihood of antisocial behaviour or juvenile delinquency (Thornberry et al., 2001). However, emotional neglect also increases the risk of mental disorders, such as affective disorders, eating disorders, dissociative disorders, personality disorders and addictions. The experience of neglecting increased stress leads to a crisis and requires appropriate support measures. Therefore, it is crucial to properly recognise the situation in which young people may find themselves in a difficult situation. In such cases, external help is often necessary to enable young people and their families to cope with the crisis. There is undoubtedly a need to re-examine current definitions of neglect in light of age-related differences and perspectives and to understand better the specific needs of young people who experience neglect.

Chapter 9

Emotional neglect in childhood

Perspectives from many years later

Study of adults' views of their experience of emotional neglect

The objectives of the study reported in this chapter were as follows: (1) identifying patterns of emotional and relational functioning in adulthood among individuals who experienced emotional neglect in childhood. Emotional neglect was defined as the misalignment of parental behaviours with children's emotional needs at different developmental stages; (2) tracing the consequences of emotional neglect dependent on the age at which it began; and (3) investigating the forms of emotional neglect experienced by children. Additionally, we explored the perception of physical pain in individuals who experienced emotional neglect. Here, emotional neglect is viewed as a phenomenon that can generate so-called social pain (see Chapter 3; Eisenberger & Lieberman, 2004), which refers to the sensation of physical pain occurring without injury or tissue damage but through mechanisms involving disruptions in relationships with significant others (rejection, exclusion, unfair treatment or relational losses).

Participants

Forty adult participants were recruited for the study reported here. All participants were involved in a larger Polish quantitative study on pain perception and stress response in relation to self-esteem and social pain. Individuals who indicated on the recruitment form for the larger study that they had experienced chronic social pain in childhood received a parallel invitation to participate in an additional interview at the end of the main study. The inclusion criteria for the smaller study were to be greater than 18 years, with experience of emotional neglect in childhood, absence of psychotic symptoms, and consent to participate in the study. 40 participants met these criteria. The adequacy of the sample size was based on guidelines for qualitative research (Marshall et al., 2013). A descriptive characterisation of the study 40 participants is presented in Table 9.1.

DOI: 10.4324/9781032621203-9

Table 9.1 Descriptive characteristics of participants in the smaller study

Participants' descriptives ($n = 40$)	
Age [*M* (SD)]	29.12 (10.74)
Gender [*n* (%)]	
Female	26 (65.0)
Male	13 (32.5)
Non-binary	1 (2.5)
Age of onset of experiencing emotional neglect [*n* (%)]	
Infancy	5 (12.5)
1–3 years	11 (27.5)
4–6 years	14 (35.0)
7–12 years	6 (15.0)
Adolescence	4 (10.0)

Procedure

The participants first underwent the procedures outlined in the main study, which involved assessing pain perception and stress response in situations threatening to self-esteem (for a full description of this part of the study, see Wojtyna et al., 2024). In this segment of the study, pain thresholds (the intensity level at which participants reported the sensation of pain) and pain tolerance thresholds (the intensity level deemed "unbearable" by participants) were determined. Pain perception and tolerance were assessed using thermal stimuli generated by a TSA-II neurosensory analyser (Medoc, Ramat Yishay, Israel). A 30 × 30 mm thermode was attached to the forearm of the non-dominant upper limb, and the thermode was gradually heated from 30 to 50.5°C at a rate of 1.5°C per second. The participants were instructed to press a button on a remote control when the heat sensation became painful (pain threshold) and when the pain became unbearable (pain tolerance threshold). Pressing the button immediately stopped the heat generation and rapidly cooled the thermode to the baseline temperature. The generated stimuli were entirely safe for the participants, and they could terminate the experiment at any time. This study was approved by the Research Ethics Committee of the University of Silesia in Katowice.

In the smaller the study, semi-structured, one-on-one interviews were conducted with the 40 participants. The choice of one-on-one interviews was based on the possibility of discussing sensitive topics in a safe environment, which participants might not be willing to disclose in focus group settings. The interviews were conducted by one of the authors of this book (EW), a researcher, a psychiatrist, and a psychotherapist. The interviews took place in an office at the university building, were recorded, and were subsequently transcribed with simultaneous anonymisation. All data that could potentially identify participants were removed from the transcripts. Participants received monetary compensation for their time, amounting to approximately USD 25. After the interview, participants were provided with answers to all their questions and, if needed, advice and information on how to obtain help for reported issues.

During the approximately one-hour conversation, participants were asked open-ended questions concerning the following areas: (1) what caregiver behaviours they associated with emotional neglect, (2) the age at which they began experiencing emotional neglect and how it progressed over their life course, (3) how they experience their emotionality, (4) how they function in close relationships and (5) how they regulate their emotional tension. The focus was on participants' subjective experiences. The responses were further detailed through additional questions. At the end of the interview, participants were given the opportunity to add any content that they deemed significant.

Analysis

We utilised an instrumental case study approach (Stake, 1997) that focused on a detailed and in-depth understanding of several selected cases to explore the broader issue of emotional neglect. The data analysis was conducted in two stages. First, an internal case analysis was performed, during which each case was comprehensively and exhaustively reconstructed (Merriam, 2009). Second, a cross-case analysis was conducted to identify the leading thematic issues that emerged from individual case studies. In categorising the obtained data, we aimed to select the most illustrative and compelling (critical cases), where the examined processes or experiences were clearly revealed, as well as the most illustrative (sensitive cases), which best exemplified the findings of the study. Following Flick's (2011) assumptions, sample selection was extended to present the research results. This was intended to not only gain knowledge and understanding of a single case but also to comprehend the issue of emotional neglect in broader terms.

Results

The study included 40 Polish individuals aged 18 to 40 years (mean age, 29 years), comprising 26 women (F), 13 men (M), and one non-binary person (NB). The majority of participants (75%) experienced emotional neglect by the age of 6 years, with 40% having such experiences between the ages of 0–3 years. Only three participants reported improvements in their relationships with caregivers during adolescence (in two cases, the parents underwent psychotherapy; in one case, the participant's mother formed a relationship with a new partner who was emotionally supportive and created a good relationship with the mother). For the remaining participants, emotional neglect persisted at various levels throughout their lives. The analysis revealed the following themes: (a) Different Faces of Emotional Neglect, (b) Emotional Turmoil versus Numbness, (c) Complete Loss of Self versus Cold Distance, (d) Punishment for Evil and (e) Numbing and Short Fuse for Pain (Table 9.2).

Table 9.2 Summary of main themes and subthemes from the interviews

Themes	Subthemes
Different faces of emotional neglect	*Emotional absence of a parent;* *High standards that do not match the child's age and needs;* *Excess extracurricular activities and excessive care*
Emotional turmoil versus numbness	Emotion regulation. Emotional sensitivity and vulnerability; Fragmented Self.
Complete loss of Self versus cold distance	Self-sacrifice.
Punishment for evil	Self-harm/self-aggression; Dissociations
Numbing and short fuse for pain	Level of awareness of pain (pain threshold); Pain tolerance

Different faces of emotional neglect

The emotional neglect described by participants revolved around three main themes: (1) emotional absence of the parent, (2) high standards misaligned with the child's age and needs and (3) an excess of extracurricular activities, or overprotection. The emotional absence of the parent was typically due to a lack of time for the child (too much work, being away from home, illness, addiction) and not listening to what the child wanted to share with the parent, as in the examples below.

Participant 28 (Female, 40 years): "I remember my mother was constantly at work, working two jobs because my father couldn't work after his accident in the mine, and most of their money went towards paying off debts. My mom never had the time to talk, and sometimes she would fall asleep while I was telling her something important to me. I couldn't talk to my father at all. Apparently, when I was little, he was full of life, but I only remember him staring at the TV and grumbling under his breath for me to leave him alone".

Participant 38 (Male, 18 years): "My father was almost never home. He either worked abroad or went out with his buddies. I think my mom couldn't handle it because, for as long as I can remember, she smoked funny-smelling

> cigarettes. You couldn't have a serious conversation with her then. It was only later that I found out it was marijuana".

The most commonly cited reason for the lack of time for the child, especially when discussing matters important to the child (sometimes perceived by parents as trivial), was work. Typically, caregivers worked long hours or their jobs required travel away from home. In seven cases, participants pointed to the issue of parents working afternoon or night shifts, which made it impossible to have contact with parents after returning from school. In three cases, the emotional absence of parents was related to the illness, death, or disability of the participants' siblings. In four cases, the participants associated their parents' lack of time with sports and training commitments.

Half of the participants highlighted the harmful use of psychoactive substances by their parents, which hindered the emotional connection between the child and parent. The most common substance used by caregivers was alcohol (39%); in 20% of cases, it was drugs (marijuana and, less frequently, psychostimulants), and in one case, a parent's addiction to opioid painkillers. This is consistent with earlier studies by Yaghoubi-Doust (2013) and Kelleher et al. (1994), which found a significant positive correlation between parents' behaviour towards their children and emotional neglect.

In 29 cases, the participants indicated that at least one of their caregivers set high standards that were not aligned with the child's age and needs. Most often, these demands were related to grades received in school. For 11 participants, parents had high expectations related to the child's achievements in competitions and contests (sports, music, academic contests), and in six participants, parents expected perfect household management from children in preschool and early school years. Conversations about parental expectations and the results achieved by participants were often the main, and in the case of eight participants, the only topic of discussion with the child, as in the examples below.

P7 (Female, 24 years): "When I messed up at a singing contest because I forgot the words to the second verse, I saw my dad turn completely red. I ran off the stage. I was perhaps six years old, in kindergarten. He grabbed me firmly by the hand and quickly led me out of the building. I couldn't keep up with him. And he just kept muttering, not even looking at me, 'such a shame, such a shame...'"

P19 (Female, 35 years): "The only thing I remember from school was my mom going through my grades. When I was in elementary school, she kept saying, 'why a five and not a six?' [In the Polish education system, fives are very good and sixes are excellent, given for outstanding achievement – author's note]. Then someone told my mom she shouldn't do that. She stopped commenting, but her expression said it all. When I brought home a lower, but still passing grade, she wouldn't speak to me for several days".

The third most common identified source of emotional neglect was the excess of organised extracurricular activities for the child or excessive parental concern:

P2 (Female, 38 years):   "I know my parents had a lot of problems with me when I was little [the participant was born with a serious heart defect – author's note]. However, even when I was healthy, they were constantly worried that something might happen to me. As a result, I couldn't run around with other kids and was banned from sports. But I wanted to. I really wanted to participate in the PE! However, the worst part was that they had to follow me everywhere. Even on my first date, my mom walked me to the cinema. I wanted to disappear. It was so embarrassing…"

P24 (Female, 26 years):   "I never had time for myself, to do nothing. After school, I went to English and Spanish classes or piano or tennis. On the weekends, I went horseback riding. My vacations were always filled with themed camps from the first day to the last day. We constantly travelled to different places. It was supposedly fun because I got to do things other kids could only dream of, but I felt best when I was sick and could stay in bed".

Participants in this area emphasised the lack of time for their own initiatives. They often feared opposing their parents ("because how do you say you don't want to do these fantastic things"), not wanting to disappoint or upset them. Each participant in this group was involved in at least three different types of extracurricular activities, occupying at least 4 hours every day. Statements such as, "my parents worked hard so I could develop, I can't be ungrateful", were common. Parents justified their behaviour by saying that, "you need a good start" and "you can't waste opportunities".

Ten participants identified excessive extracurricular activities as a source of emotional neglect. Six of them have difficulties in adulthood with independently planning their activities and "don't know what they want in life". The remaining four participants have problems with resting, e.g., "when I have some free time and could lie in bed longer on weekends, I immediately feel guilty that I'm wasting time and it would be better to do something useful" (**P4, Female, 35 years**).

Emotional turmoil versus numbness

Most participants (35 individuals) had difficulty understanding and expressing their anger. It is worth mentioning that many children who have experienced emotional neglect have difficulty regulating their emotions (Zhang et al., 2022). Participants' beliefs about this emotion were dominated by thoughts such as, "you shouldn't get angry", "anger is bad", or "if I show I'm angry, I'll get punished". Most often, participants became angry at themselves when anger arose and took one of two paths: either they suppressed their anger or engaged in self-harm. Those who chose to suppress their emotions more frequently complained about various somatic ailments.

For other emotions, the necessity to suppress them was also common. Fear was often trivialised by parents, or participants were shamed by their parents when they were afraid (**P35, Female, 26 years**): "My mother always shrugged and said I was being hysterical"). Curiosity was considered bothersome and unwelcome (**P39, Male, 22 years**): "I constantly heard that curiosity is the first step to hell. And I didn't want to go to hell"). Sadness was devalued (**P16, Female, 21 years**): "My parents always tried to cheer me up, saying: come on, smile, look at the beautiful weather"). More than half of the participants (26 individuals) declared that they were extremely sensitive, that, "emotions overwhelm them", "emotions are unbearable", "a storm in the head that's impossible to manage". Seven participants explicitly described themselves as highly sensitive individuals. At the same time, all of these individuals held the belief that experiencing such emotions indicated, "weakness and an inability to cope with life".

On the other hand, 10 participants stated that they, "feel nothing":

P18 (Male, 21 years):	"I was never afraid of anything. People would panic before tests or exams, but I was always relaxed. I do extreme sports and have never felt fear".
P30 (Female, 30 years):	"I know I love my girlfriend, but it's all in my head. I don't really understand what it feels like to feel love. I read about it in books and hear about it from people, even from my girlfriend, but I don't feel it. It's the same when I have sex. I don't feel elation, I'm not swept away".

This emotional numbness in eight participants out of the ten individuals who reported this issue was generalised across the emotional spectrum—both positive and negative affect. For the remaining two, the numbness included only positive emotions and anger.

Fragmented Self

Thirty-two participants (80%), including all who experienced emotional neglect in their early years of life before starting school, reported symptoms typical of a dissociative personality structure (Nijenhuis & van der Hart, 2011). In this context, a person's personality is divided into at least two subsystems (dissociative parts of the personality) characterised by insufficient integration, a dynamic nature, excessive stability, and a rudimentary first-person perspective. Among the participants, dissociative parts of the personality most often switched sequentially, with one part typically being more stable and dominant, especially in those who experienced neglect at the earliest stages of life (0–3 years). The switching of parts was most commonly triggered by three categories of stimuli: (1) strong emotions; (2) facial expressions of negative emotions by people interacting with the participant; (3) deprived physiological needs:

P14 (Female, 25 years): "I often feel like I'm not myself, like something switches tracks in my mind. It's very bothersome. Sometimes, when I'm really excited about something, suddenly this wedge comes into my head, like an on-off switch: my emotion suddenly changes from joy, like when I was about to go to a concert, to a terrible sense of guilt, and I don't even know why".

P22 (Female, 24 years): "I have a really good relationship. Normally, I feel very safe in it. But when I see my girlfriend's gaze wander or when she's sad, this wave of warmth washes over me, from my stomach through my whole body. And it's a horrible feeling. I curl up inside. Immediately, I think, 'it's my fault, I must have done something wrong.' It takes me a long time to recover".

P4 (Female, 35 years): "I'm usually like a battering ram, like a robot. Super efficient and indestructible. However, if I forget to eat regularly or lose sleep – which happened a lot in college – suddenly, this helplessness and weakness would switch on. I would then spiral into a void. I could curl up under a blanket for hours and not want to live. Eventually, the familiar voice kicks in, telling me 'you're a lazy bum, get to work.' And I finally get up…"

Complete loss of Self versus cold distance

In the area of forming close relationships, participants exhibited one of the following tendencies: either they did not engage in close relationships

(10 individuals), which was also demonstrated in earlier studies by Klein and Kuiper (2006), they completely self-sacrificed in relationships (16 individuals), or they alternated between distancing themselves and becoming completely absorbed in relationships (10 individuals):

P5 (Non-binary, 19 years): "When I fall in love, I disappear. There's only that person. I breathe them, I live them".

P9 (Male, 27 years): "I've never been in a relationship. It's not that I avoid people. I seek contact. However, if someone tries to flirt with me, I will shut down completely and immediately withdraw. My whole being tells me it's not for me".

P33 (Female, 29 years): "I can't build a lasting relationship. Something's not right. I keep ending up with the wrong guys. In the beginning, it's amazing! He's amazing, perfect. I fall head over heels. I quickly want more and more from this relationship. I give everything. However, after a few months, I'm left alone. First, everything hurts; I cry from the pain, and it completely takes me out of life. I want to die. Then, for the next few months, I don't even want to go out. It's not that I have any prejudice. Men just become indifferent to me. They become invisible".

Punishment for evil

In the face of experiencing high levels of stress and/or emotional tension, participants revealed the following coping patterns: (1) self-harm/self-aggression; (2) dissociation; (3) avoidance; and (4) aggression, with the first two being the most strongly represented. Self-harm was reported by 36 participants and was most often undertaken in situations associated with anger and helplessness:

P3 (Female, 34 years): "The first time I cut myself was when I told my mom that my father took my comic book collection and gave it to his daughter from his second marriage. I was 13 years old then. I know it's just comics, but they were MY comics, and when I felt bad, I could look through them for hours. And he just took them without asking. I told my mom, and she just said that I was big and shouldn't be making a fuss. That night, I took a pocketknife and made dozens of cuts on my forearm".

P31 (Male, 37 years):   "I used to hit my fists against the rough wall of the garage. The first time? I was maybe in sixth grade [about 12 years old – author's note], when the boys from the sports club where I trained were bullying me. They called me a 'sissy'. I didn't want to go there, I was scared. I begged my father to let me quit. He just said that I surely didn't mean it and walked out in the middle of my sentence, saying he had an important meeting with a neighbour. When he left me alone, something hit me–an emptiness, but also a strange impulse. I realized it when my hand was already bloody".

The above statements are consistent with the findings of studies conducted by Cassels et al. (2018), Nemati et al. (2020), and Hou et al. (2023), which showed that in dysfunctional families, where emotional neglect is more frequent, the risk of non-suicidal self-injury increases.

Participants usually engaged in self-harm at home, most often in a way that other household members would not notice. Inflicting pain on themselves was described by participants as a way to alleviate psychological suffering, providing temporary "relief" or a sense of "calm". Analysing the motives driving participants to self-harm, the most common reasons were emotion regulation (75%) and self-punishment (64%). For 11 participants (30.5%), the motive for self-harm was the desire to identify with a peer group/subculture in which they felt accepted. Ten participants associated self-harm with the desire to "disappear". For six participants, self-harm served the purpose of attracting parental attention, and for two participants, self-harm was a way to avoid hurting others (parent or sibling).

The motive of self-punishment was most often associated with feelings of having disappointed or let down a parent. Participants interpreted their behaviours as wrong but primarily revealed a perception of themselves as bad individuals. They associated badness with something that deserved punishment or needed to be atoned for through pain:

P12 (Female, 40 years):   "Whenever I broke a house rule and did something forbidden, it was unbearable afterward. Most often, this happened when I forgot myself and went out with my friends. And if I came back a bit later, I would see that my sick mother had cleaned the apartment herself and was lying down, moaning in pain [a disabled mother with OCD about cleanliness, raising the participant alone – author's note]. And it was supposed to be my job. I felt like the worst scum, an ingrate. A terrible person".

P27 (Female, 35 years):   "It's the feeling when you know you're disappointing everyone around you, when you know you're just a bad person, that you messed everything up again. That you don't deserve to live".

Four participants who never engaged in self-harm reported experiencing emotional neglect only during adolescence. The others, who experienced neglect earlier, typically began self-harming during adolescence. This aligns with the findings of Hou et al. (2023), who noted that non-suicidal self-injury often begins during adolescence.

Numbing and short fuse for pain

In the area of physical pain perception, interview responses were compared with the results obtained by participants in the main study, which measured pain thresholds and tolerance using thermal stimuli. Participants primarily highlighted two seemingly contradictory aspects of pain perception. On one hand, most participants (30 individuals) stated that they frequently experienced nonspecific pain (migraines, back pain, joint pain, pain in areas of old injuries), often needed physiotherapy (most commonly related to spinal pain), and were patients of neurologists and orthopaedists. On the other hand, they sometimes fail to notice injuries or, in the case of self-harm, practically do not feel pain:

P23 (Male, 25 years):   "Sometimes I wouldn't realize I was hurt until I noticed my clothes were bloody. But on the other hand, at the dentist, it hurts when he just touches my teeth with a tool. It's embarrassing".

P40 (Female, 27 years):   "I'm only twenty-seven, but I'm so sickly. Everything hurts, I'm constantly on painkillers, but they hardly help. But the funniest thing is, when I gave birth, it didn't hurt at all. And I was threatened with this childbirth before".

Emotional neglect and pain thresholds

In the study of pain thresholds and pain tolerance using thermal stimuli, the results were analysed in the context of the age at which participants began experiencing emotional neglect. The results show a similar level of pain tolerance across all participants. However, for pain thresholds, the highest thresholds were observed in participants who experienced emotional neglect during infancy, while the lowest thresholds were found in those who experienced neglect only during adolescence. This configuration of pain threshold and pain tolerance indicates that individuals who experienced emotional neglect very early in life have a very small window between the moment they become aware of the pain and the moment the pain becomes unbearable.

A statistically significant negative correlation was observed between the age at which participants began experiencing emotional neglect and their pain threshold. The younger the participants were when they experienced neglect, the higher their reported pain threshold. No significant correlation was found between the age of onset of emotional neglect and pain tolerance threshold.

Emotional neglect as a significant source of problems in adulthood

The analysis of the interviews and the results of the pain threshold study suggests several inferences. First, there appears to be a similarity between the dynamics of emotional experiences and pain perception, as demonstrated by the quantitative study using the physical thermal stimulus. A common feature seems to be the elevated threshold for becoming aware of painful or emotional sensations. Most participants exhibited a kind of numbness or detachment. In the main study, of which the additional interviews presented here were a part, it was observed that individuals who experienced chronic social pain (i.e., feelings of rejection in relationships, unfair treatment, feelings of loss in relationships) and simultaneously had fragile self-esteem, experienced threats to the Self in a specific manner (Wojtyna et al., 2024). These individuals showed the highest pain threshold among all participants, and after exposure to the threat of rejection, an increase in pain tolerance threshold was noted, along with elevated cortisol levels and the longest-lasting cortisol response to stress. This indicates that such individuals may be prone to overlooking significant pain symptoms, and a prolonged stress response could expose them to conditions resulting from chronic stress. The interview analysis also points to a tendency to develop a dissociative personality structure and disturbances in recognising boundaries in close relationships. An important observation from the study is the relationship between the severity and type of symptoms experienced by adults and the age at which emotional neglect by parents began. This topic will be explored further in Chapter 10.

Finally, the interviews highlighted new phenomena in the area of emotional neglect, such as excessive parental concern for the child's development and the attempt to take advantage of all opportunities that parents believe could be beneficial for the child. It emerged that excessive extracurricular activities and over-involvement by parents in their children's lives were significant factors impairing the quality of life of the participants.

Chapter 10

Taking care of neglected needs

Protecting children from the effects of emotional neglect is crucial in preventing mental health disorders, and potential self-harm, attempted suicide and death in adulthood. The phenomenon by which emotional neglect plays a significant role has been thoroughly described in earlier chapters. This has allowed for the identification of various risk factors and protective factors at different levels, from the individual characteristics of parents, children, and adolescents, through family relationships, to broader social and cultural contexts. Recognising risk and protective factors is key to creating effective prevention programmes and interventions in cases of emotional neglect in children and adolescents, as well as in preventing possible long-term and intergenerational consequences (Strathearn et al., 2009). Additionally, the understanding that different types of childhood trauma (including emotional neglect) may have intergenerational effects has significant implications for the creation of public policies, family support programmes, and therapeutic interventions.

The negative impact of emotional neglect in childhood on mental health can be long-lasting, whereas positive experiences, which may be provided by teachers or caregivers in institutions where children and adolescents are cared for, can help mitigate these effects (Glickman et al., 2021). Furthermore, identifying potential protective factors, especially those that can be incorporated at early stages of development, can help promote the mental health of children and youth who have experienced emotional neglect.

Human development occurs through the continuous interaction of internal factors related to an individual's personal resources (both genetic and developed in earlier developmental phases), and external factors related to the quality of the environment in which a person lives (diversity, opportunity to satisfy needs, and support for development). In this chapter, we attempt to integrate observations about the symptoms and effects of emotional neglect in children and adolescents and discuss preventive and treatment possibilities.

Emotionality and emotional neglect

Emotional neglect is primarily understood as a lack of alignment between the external environment and emotional needs of the child which are

DOI: 10.4324/9781032621203-10

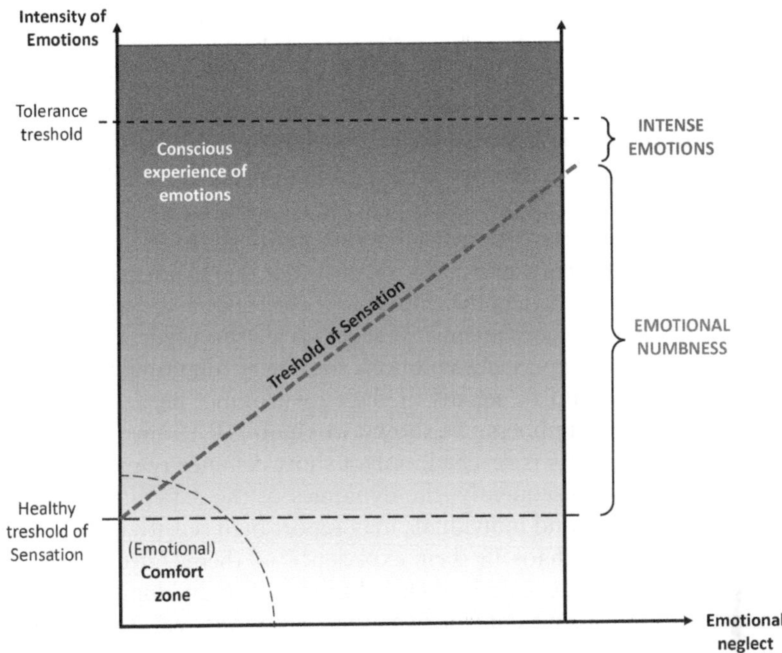

Figure 10.1 Hypothetical model of human emotionality related to emotional neglect experienced in childhood.

characteristic of various stages of human development. An appropriate match between external conditions and internal needs enables effective accomplishment of developmental tasks. In the absence of such an alignment, even with the exceptionally broad internal resources of children, one can expect that their development will not proceed properly.

Figure 10.1 presents a hypothetical model of human emotionality related to emotional neglect experienced in childhood.

In healthy conditions, individuals have access to the full spectrum of emotional experiences, both qualitatively (type of emotion) and quantitatively (intensity of emotions). In the area marked in the figure as the Comfort Zone, human needs are met, and thus, no emotional signals reach their consciousness that would prompt them to take action. This does not imply a lack of access to emotions. If a person makes an effort and closely examines their experience, they will be able to accurately determine their state. Above the healthy threshold of sensation, or rather, awareness of feeling emotions, a clear message about a particular emotion and/or need emerges in an individual's mind. Initially, it is a weak signal, so it does not disrupt current functioning, but as emotions intensify, it becomes increasingly difficult to maintain focus on current activities. There is a strong need to respond to emotional signals. Finally, upon reaching the tolerance threshold, discomfort is so intense that immediate action is necessary, as it becomes unbearable. Here, two pathways emerge: the first is the immediate fulfilment of the need (which may either occur in a socially acceptable way or the opposite) or dissociation (as in Post-traumatic Stress Disorder). In people with a secure attachment style, there is a vast space between the threshold of sensation and the emotional tolerance threshold, providing individuals with ample ability to act and calmly seek solutions.

Individuals who have experienced emotional neglect are likely to experience a disruption in this pattern. We suggest that due to experiencing strong tensions, often from infancy, the threshold for emotional awareness is raised (through dissociation mechanisms). If such a situation occurs, the individual will not consciously experience emotions for a very long time (and thus will not be able to respond to signals of their own unmet needs), leading to a state of emotional numbness. As shown in Figure 10.1, once the threshold of emotional awareness is reached, only a short distance remains to the tolerance threshold. Consequently, the dynamics of the experienced emotions become very intense, and individuals may report high sensitivity, intolerance of emotions, and/or chaos in their experience of them. Often, there is no longer enough space to calmly seek solutions, so individuals begin to act impulsively, often losing control over their emotions (e.g., experiencing a panic attack or impulsively destroying their surroundings). Such situations often lead individuals to a state of "unbearability", which – especially in the presence of continued emotional neglect from the environment (indicating a lack of safety) – means a further tendency to dissociate and a further need to defensively raise the threshold of emotional awareness.

We suggest that the earlier the experience of emotional neglect, the greater the shortening of the distance between the threshold of emotional awareness and the tolerance threshold one can expect. However, unlike typical emotional disorders (where the threshold of emotional awareness remains physiologically low and only the emotional tolerance threshold is lowered), in neglected children, not only is the range of experienced emotions shortened but it is also raised to the upper registers of the scale (see Figure 10.1). However, emotions are necessary to effectively satisfy important needs. Quickly and healthily reading emotional signals allows one to engage in behaviours that, at a low energy cost, maintain comfort while remaining balanced in both external and internal life.

In addition to signalling needs, emotions play an important role in establishing boundaries in relationships. They indicate when something is happening in a relationship and they are alert when boundaries are violated. For individuals who have experienced emotional neglect and an elevated threshold of emotional awareness, recognising boundaries is consequently difficult, and building close relationships is fraught with the risk of failure and abuse. Therefore, there may be occurrences of exploitation and abuse as well as crossing the boundaries of others (often with good intentions).

In both cases, there is no conscious mutual negotiation or building of new quality in the relationship. Instead, the relationship is likely to be shaped by a submissive-dominance dimension. The Self of one party will have to yield to the Self of the other; otherwise, an unbearable conflict will occur. Such functioning can be observed, for example, in borderline personality disorders (Steele et al., 2019; Vermetten & Spiegel, 2014).

Development of self from infancy to adolescence

The issue of respecting an individual's boundaries within their surroundings, as well as the ability to signal when these boundaries are crossed, are important factors in the development of the Self. Our understanding of the development of the Self in children experiencing emotional neglect is shown in Figure 10.2.

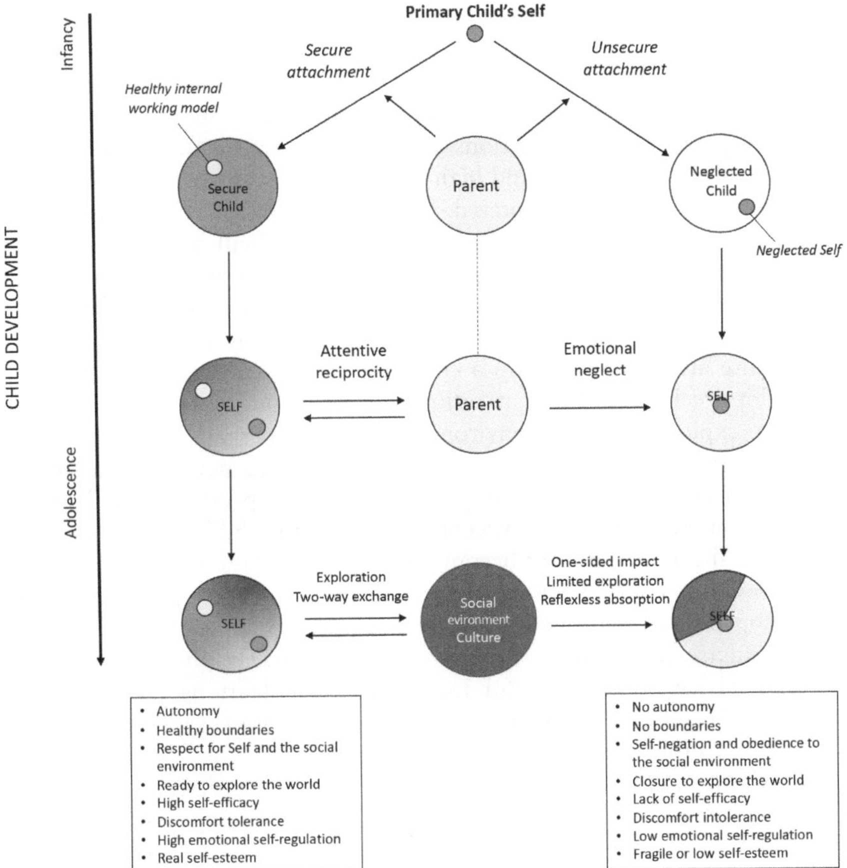

Figure 10.2 Development of Self from infancy to adolescence.

When children are born, they are completely dependent on their caregivers and lack the tools to defend themselves and their boundaries. Depending on how the relationship between caregivers and the child develops, either a secure or insecure attachment style emerges. In the former case, the child's Self, which we understand as the individual's autonomous and unique characteristics, can develop without obstacles. Feeling safe and having a stable background, children will willingly explore their surroundings while maintaining their own uniqueness. Simultaneously, a healthy internalised representation of caregivers (internal working model) is formed in the child's psyche, laying the groundwork for further development. As children progress through childhood and adolescence, they gather experiences through close, mutually attentive relationships with adults and the socio-cultural environment, which can be subjected to increasingly deep reflection. This allows them to gradually and safely shape their mature identity, which is capable of reconciling their autonomous and social needs. The internal working model will be a clear, though not unyieldingly strict and indisputable, core of the young person's moral principles. In turn, their autonomous Self will be accepted and respected by the environment (increasingly extending beyond the family), which will see in the young person a new quality that enriches the social group. In such conditions, the young person has the chance to build healthy realistic self-esteem and high self-efficacy, or the belief that they can cope despite obstacles encountered. Experiencing difficult emotions will not block such an individual; despite discomfort, they will be able to develop their values, seek the meaning of life, and explore the world, including the area of close relationships, thanks to a healthy perception of boundaries.

However, if emotional neglect by caregivers leads to the development of an insecure attachment style in a child, the individual Self will not be able to develop freely. The child's attention will not be directed towards free and reflective exploration of the environment but will perhaps attempt to draw the attention of those around them. This often means developing a strategy of hypersensitivity and uncovering the needs and expectations of the social environment. Fulfilling these expectations allows the child to "earn" its place in the social group. The Self becomes filled with values and duties dictated by the environment, while the child's original unique predispositions remain undeveloped and often dissociated. Such a person will not be autonomous; their existence (place in the group) will depend solely on what they do – on the basis of obedience – for the environment (earning merit and self-sacrifice). Their Self is shaped by rules adopted directly and without any adaptation to the individual's autonomous predispositions. Such individuals often exhibit high intolerance to discomfort, limited insight into their own emotionality, and consequently, difficulties in maintaining healthy boundaries in close relationships. In case of discrepancies between principles prevailing in the family and the social environment (e.g., in groups where the child functions outside the family), one can expect "switching" between these principles in an "on-off" mechanism. This is consistent with the concept of dissociative personality structure (Nijenhuis & van der Hart, 2011), as well as with the schema mode theory developed within schema therapy (Young et al., 2003). In such cases, self-esteem is expected to develop in one of the two directions: low or fragile. We speak of fragile self-esteem when there is a discrepancy between explicit and implicit self-esteem. Explicit self-esteem refers to self-aware beliefs about an individual's own worth. Implicit self-esteem is understood as the influence of self-attitude on the evaluation of objects related and unrelated to the self (Greenwald & Banaji, 1995). This type of self-esteem develops based on childhood experiences (Bosson et al., 2003). Low implicit self-esteem is associated with greater susceptibility to external cues such as image evaluations, clear successes in undertaken activities, and explicit signals of acceptance from the environment (Jordan & Zeigler-Hill, 2013; Wojtyna et al., 2024). Often, individuals with low implicit self-esteem attempt to protect their own worth by implementing compensatory strategies (Wojtyna et al., 2024). In such cases, an individual may achieve many successes, have many contacts, and even hold high beliefs about their worth in terms of explicit self-esteem, yet their self-esteem remains fragile. This means that any threat to the self will provoke the activation of protective strategies for the Self (avoidance, compensation, attack, etc.) (Wojtyna et al., 2023, 2024). In such cases, the individual's attention is always directed towards searching for threats, which means chronic stress on the one hand, but also insufficient processing and analysis of data in neuronal mentalisation circuits (see Chapter 3). These processes will foster further development of those parts of the Self that have been imposed on the individual through harsh parental and sociocultural influences (the yellow and red areas in the representation of the Self in Figure 10.2), while the neglected original Self will undergo further marginalisation and attempts to diminish this part of oneself. However, this time, the perpetrators of neglect are the individuals themselves. This leads to self-neglect, and in extreme cases, can even lead to self-annihilation.

The earlier the originally autonomous Self of the child is ignored, the greater disturbances in the structure of the Self can be expected. Personality undergoes fragmentation into dissociative parts (Nijenhuis & van der Hart, 2011) or schema modes (Young et al., 2003). When the level of emotional neglect reaches the level of emotional trauma the resulting schema modes may operate in a separate manner which may resemble dissociative identity disorders (DID) (Krause-Utz et al., 2017; Nijenhuis & van der Hart, 2011; Vermetten and Spiegel, 2014). In cases where the environmental reinforcement of schema modes is strong, one (or sometimes several) of them may begin to dominate and function relatively stable for a long time. In such cases, the individual functions coherently and only strong stimuli can cause a switch to another mode. However, this seemingly stable functioning in one mode is not healthy for the individual. The resulting chronic deprivation of needs constitutes chronic stress and mental tension, which are risk factors for the development of mental and psychosomatic disorders. According to our hypotheses, the tension experienced may be poorly understood by the individual owing to elevated thresholds for becoming aware of emotions. In dissociative disorders, abnormalities have been demonstrated in the activity of central nervous system structures, such as the amygdala, insula, and prefrontal cortex (Krause-Utz et al., 2017). These changes in brain structure activation may account for difficulties in adequately receiving and interpreting emotional signals.

Towards healthier emotionality and integration of Self

The hypotheses presented above – about the elevated thresholds of emotional awareness and the existence of emotional numbness zones, as well as the possibility of personality fragmentation under the influence of emotional neglect trauma – prompt us to inquire about the possibilities for correcting this situation. Certainly, more hopeful scenarios exist when emotional neglect occur later in a child's life. In these cases, the integrated part of the Self is larger and stronger, and access to and communication with dissociative parts of the personality is easier. These parts should also have access to more mature mechanisms for processing the information and interpreting the reality available to them. In cases where emotional neglect occurred very early, working on the integration of the Self will be much more challenging and may resemble working with an entire system of personality components (analogous to family therapy) rather than working one-on-one with an individual. A necessary condition for planning adequate and potentially effective help is a thorough understanding of the person's situation and an analysis of areas such as personality structure, self-image, access to emotionality, and resources available to the individual. Neglecting this understanding could lead to premature and misguided forms of assistance. Such actions pose a risk of intensifying the stress on the beneficiaries of our efforts.

Analysing a person's life-line in terms of meeting their emotional needs, which differ in various developmental periods, allows us to gauge the level of dissociative fragmentation of personality. At the same time, we gain insights into self-image. It then becomes easier to discern whether the individual integrates both their unique autonomous areas and the influences related to functioning in significant social groups – family, educational systems, and peer groups – into their Self.

Locating difficult experiences along the life-line helps determine whether an individual has reached important milestones in the physiological development of humans. If gaps are identified, the expected consequences of an individual's functioning can be considered. The right-thumb desire to identify and medicalise all problems present in an individual may lead us to want to correct everything. Thus, there are effective and useful therapeutic methods at our disposal. However, remembering the vicious cycle of the right-thumb understanding of health illustrated in Figure 1 of Chapter 2 of this book, we must be aware of the risk of generating further problems with interventions originally intended to be corrective. To protect against excessive interventions, it is advisable to situate the problems of people with experiences of emotional neglect within the diathesis-stress model (Scheeringa, 2021). This model assumes that psychopathological symptoms result from improper processing of information by the responsible neural circuits. However, the functioning of these neural circuits depends on the interaction between biological factors (diathesis) and the stressor load (stress).

From the diathesis viewpoint, it is necessary to consider changes in the brain structures and neural circuits responsible for processing emotions, building empathic relationships, and mentalisation (see Chapter 3). In individuals with experiences of emotional neglect, the functioning of these brain areas may be disrupted. This increases the risk of decompensation and emergence of psychopathological symptoms when exposed to stress.

Stress can be generated by various sources. First, emotional neglect itself may still be present and affect the individual as a strong stressor. Daily problems, including those arising from difficulties with relationships, are another source of stress. Additionally, strong current sociocultural influences, such as right-thumb maximisation, can also be stressors. The effect of stress on neural circuits in the diathesis-stress model is moderated by personality factors and support resources. From the personality theory viewpoint, the structure of the personality and attachment styles should be considered. In individuals with experiences of emotional neglect, the personality structure may be dissociated, and numerous problems in coping with everyday challenges may be rooted in this dissociation (Nijenhuis & van der Hart, 2011). An insecure attachment style and the resulting strategies of functioning in relationships can make a person more susceptible to the effects of stressors. These factors can significantly intensify the importance of stressors in the diathesis-stress model. Social support is an important moderator. Individuals who experience emotional neglect often find it difficult to build healthy and supportive interpersonal relationships. However, social support can significantly reduce the negative consequences of excessive stress (Xiong et al., 2022). Social resources are not only a buffer for stress, but also an important factor in the broad primary and secondary prevention of emotional neglect.

Social resources as a protective factor against emotional neglect and its consequences

Dunn et al. (2002) found that the social resources of parents, children and adolescents are important protective factors that moderate the impact of neglect. These include support groups for parents, meetings, and workshops that help parents cope with the challenges of raising children by offering emotional support and sharing experiences. Valuable options include parental counselling and coaching, which provide professional support with techniques and strategies for dealing with difficult parenting situations. It is also important to consider caregiving services – access to kindergartens, nurseries, or day care – which can relieve parents and provide them time to work, take care of their own needs, or regenerate (Ludwig & Rostain, 2009).

Assuming that parents may neglect their children because of a lack of knowledge, educational programmes that raise awareness of the consequences of neglect and offer help in parenting skills training are crucial. A particularly important element of such support for parents is training in interpersonal communication. Neglectful parents may communicate in ways that lead to feelings of loneliness, lack of support, and a lack of understanding of the child. Instead of empathetic communication (e.g., "I see you're sad, let's talk about what's bothering you"), there may be trivialisation of the child's problems and emotions ("Don't make a scene, everyone has problems"). Instead of support ("I'm with you, no matter what, we'll get through this together"), there may be rejection ("You need to manage on your own, I also had tough times and no one helped me"). Instead of recognition ("You did well, I'm proud of your effort"), there may be devaluation ("Is that all? I expected better results"). Changes in parent-child communication can be the basis for further supportive actions for the child and the entire family.

As shown in earlier chapters, for school-aged children and adolescents, in addition to the family, the influence of peer relationships becomes very important. The quality of friendships can be a potential moderator of the relationship between emotional neglect in childhood and the risk of developing mental disorders such as depression in adolescents (Dong et al., 2023). Therefore, promoting friendships as an intervention and preventive element for working with children and adolescents is emphasised. Developing programmes that support the building and maintenance of strong peer bonds can be a key element in preventing the negative consequences of emotional neglect among children and adolescents. Such interventions can significantly contribute to improving the overall mental state and provide better tools for coping in adult life.

Professional support in primary and secondary prevention of emotional neglect

Professionals, such as teachers, psychologists, educators, and healthcare workers, play a crucial role in the psychoeducation of parents or other legal guardians of children. Teachers are in an ideal position to recognise and report warning signs and indicators of neglect. In some European countries, such as Bulgaria, Croatia, Denmark, Estonia, France, Hungary, Ireland, Lithuania, Luxembourg, Poland, Romania, Slovenia, Spain, Sweden, and the United Kingdom, all professionals are legally obligated to report known or suspected cases of child neglect.

Psychoeducation should focus on the importance of responding appropriately to a child's needs and developing communication skills and techniques for dealing with stress and frustration. This highlights that protection against emotional neglect requires an integrated approach that combines early problem identification, parental psychoeducation, and professional support. It also emphasises the need to raise public awareness of the symptoms and impact of emotional abuse and neglect on mental health. It is crucial that these issues be appropriately recognised in global child protection laws and policies (Kumari, 2020). Children up to three years old are most vulnerable to abuse and neglect because they are most defenceless and have the least contact with people outside the family who might notice and intervene on behalf of the child. Therefore, protecting a child from emotional neglect should include early recognition of warning signals by doctors and others in contact with the child and its family, considering the damage it can cause (Kumari, 2020). However, it is not always possible to identify at-risk children. For example, families of high socioeconomic status may escape the attention of child protection agencies (Crittenden, 1999), especially because contemporary causes of emotional neglect may take forms resembling care (numerous extracurricular activities and overprotectiveness; see Chapter 9). It is important to distinguish between risk factors and actual harmful interactions between caregivers and children. Glaser's (2002) concept of "levels of concern", with external levels representing contexts and internal levels representing specific factors and interactions, highlights the need for professionals to collect comprehensive information and understand complex family narratives to properly identify and deal with emotional neglect.

Finally, individuals affected by emotional neglect may benefit from psychotherapeutic methods. Considering that therapeutic interventions are less often applied to neglected children, and, "there is a lack of research on its prevalence in the general population (Ylitervo et al., 2023, p. 1)". Ylitervo et al. (2023) highlighted the need for targeted psychological interventions that pay special attention to parents who have experienced childhood trauma. Addressing the past traumas of parents can be crucial in preventing the transmission of trauma to the next generation.

It is also worth noting diagnostic and therapeutic methods based on feedback. Leclère et al. (2018) demonstrated that video feedback is an effective tool for diagnosing and treating early interactions between parents and children in situations of serious emotional neglect. The use of methods such as video feedback not only helps assess the quality of the interaction between the parent and child but also serves a therapeutic support role, enabling parents to better understand and improve their responses to the needs of the child. Utilising such a tool allows for building a more conscious and sensitive parental relationship, which is crucial in countering the negative effects of emotional neglect and supporting healthy development of the child (Leclère et al., 2018).

Our analysis of a child's developmental needs and the possible mechanisms by which their significant emotional needs are unmet led us to closely examine specific possibilities for psychotherapeutic support for individuals affected by emotional neglect, as discussed below.

Returning to healthier paths through (non-right-thumb) psychotherapy

Before we look more closely at specific psychotherapeutic interventions that may be helpful, let us return to the issue of the risks associated with introducing excessive corrective actions. The diathesis-stress model clearly indicates the interactive rather than deterministic influence of biological factors and stressors on the development of mental-health problems. Therefore, we can expect that each individual will have different needs, and that the pursuit of balance may take various forms. However, interventions aimed at helping people, including psychotherapy, may be associated with increased stress. This is usually a temporary and strictly controlled state; however, it is inherent in the process of change in therapy. Thus, thoughtless assistance can exacerbate, rather than reduce, the problems faced by neglected individuals. Similarly, overprotectiveness and a tendency to maximise goals on the part of parents are often cited in this book as risk factors for children's emotional neglect. Victims of emotional neglect may also succumb to right-thumb maximisation in order to earn a noticeable place in society. What should be done?

To break free from the right-thumb pursuit of correcting all problems, it is worthwhile to reflect on the specific situation of individuals. In addition to analysing the resources available to them, their self-image, and diagnosing their personality structure, it is advisable to extend reflection to the intervention itself. We propose that all psychotherapeutic interventions discussed below should be considered from a metacognitive perspective, taking into account empirical evidence of the effectiveness of each method, and additionally considering the specific emotional needs and symptoms resulting from the emotional neglect experienced.

Analysing the proposed aid in terms of its functionality for the individual may be helpful. A functional analysis of beliefs, as in Rational Behaviour Therapy (RBT), may be useful (Wirga et al., 2020). In this cognitive-behavioural psychotherapeutic method, belief analysis is based on so-called Rules for Healthy Thinking. Inspired by these rules, we can ask the following reflective questions before undertaking the intended therapeutic intervention:

1 Is the intervention I want to undertake based on rational grounds? This does not refer to seemingly "(pseudo)scientific" grounds, but to robust empirical knowledge and a thorough analysis of potential gains and costs, which the following four questions may also help address;

2 Does the intervention I want to undertake help protect the health and life of the person it is intended to help? Does this action not expose them to chronic stress? Particular attention should be paid here to the diathesis-stress model;

3 Does the intervention I want to undertake help achieve important goals and values for that person? Do we know of these values?

4 Does the intervention I want to undertake help establish and maintain healthy relationships with others? Does it help to resolve conflicts with important individuals? Does this intervention address the emotional needs of the individual that are related to experiencing close relationships, including specific needs stemming from their attachment style and issues of experienced neglect?

5 Does the intervention I want to undertake support the psychological well-being and quality of life of that person?

According to the principles of RBT, not all Rules for Healthy Thinking need to be met; the majority may suffice. This flexibility, based on an individual's personal experience, allows decisions to be made that may be better tailored to the authentic needs of the individual. Thus, we avoid the risk of further emotional neglect of the given individual and break free from the right-thumb vicious circle that leads to the escalation of stress.

Specific issues related to emotional neglect and psychotherapeutic methods of treatment

Based on our considerations, the most significant problems requiring special attention in psychotherapy for individuals who have experienced emotional neglect are: (1) insecure attachment style; (2) dissociative personality structure; (3) dissociations; and (4) disorders of emotional regulation, including those associated with the hypothetical raising of the threshold for emotional awareness.

While attachment style is one of the most fundamental aspects of the human psyche and is thus very stable over time (e.g., Waters et al., 2000), there are reports of the potential for the development of earned secure attachment later in life in individuals with initially insecure attachments (Dansby Olufowote et al., 2020; Jańczak, 2023; Saunders et al., 2011; Zaccagnino et al., 2014). One highlighted mechanism for this change involves an individual's experiences in relationships with healthy and safe partners or other adults. The corrective behaviours of partners or other adults related to closeness can allow for the revision of attachment concepts (Johnson & Whiffen, 1999). This highlights opportunities to use psychotherapy as a means of providing such corrective experiences.

Experiencing a secure relationship with a therapist can heal in itself regardless of the psychotherapeutic approach. However, in the context of our discussions of emotional neglect, at least two aspects deserve attention. The first is the duration of this relationship and the second is the experience of emotional support. Saunders et al. (2011) demonstrated that a shift towards earned secure attachment depends on a greater number of psychotherapy hours. A longer duration of psychotherapy allows one to experience many aspects of a close relationship and its dynamics. This relates to the second aspect, which is crucial. We expect that the more authentically the therapist expresses emotions, the more efficient the process of change will occur. Consistent with our assumptions are findings of the effectiveness of emotional focused therapy (EFT) (e.g., Burgess Moser et al., 2016; Elliott & Macdonald, 2021; Harrington et al., 2021; Johnson & Whiffen, 1999) and dialectical behaviour therapy (DBT) (e.g., Fassbinder et al., 2016; Foote & Van Orden, 2016; Gupta et al., 2019) in emotional trauma. It has also been shown that a change towards secure attachment is more likely when an individual's original cognitive models of Self and others are more flexible (Johnson & Whiffen, 1999). In this case, therapeutic methods based on attachment-oriented therapy (e.g., Burgess Moser et al., 2016; Ewing et al., 2015) and acceptance and commitment therapy (ACT) (e.g., A-Tjak et al., 2020; Pohar & Argáez, 2017; Yadavaia et al., 2014) may be effective.

Another crucial mechanism leading to changes towards earned secure attachment involves experiencing emotional support from alternative individuals (Saunders et al., 2011). Here, psychotherapy can operate on two levels. The support providers can be the therapists themselves (nonspecific level), or the goal of therapy may be to strengthen the ability to obtain such support from close individuals (specific level). In the latter case, methods drawn from systematic therapy or attachment-based family therapy (Diamond et al., 2021) may be effective.

The above-mentioned methods can be helpful in implementing the factors identified by Dansby Olufowote et al. (2020), which leads to the building of earned secure attachment. The authors list several factors, including being intentional about attachment-focused change, having surrogate attachment figures, making intrapsychic changes (redefining identity and self-worth, relinquishing the victim's mentality), and making interpersonal changes (making peace with the past, revisiting caregivers with a new lens, taking small risks with trust).

In previous chapters, we repeatedly pointed out the issue of personality fragmentation and the emergence of dissociative parts of personality, or so-called schema modes. In cases where an individual with a history of emotional neglect exhibits functioning in such parts, therapeutic methods dedicated to working with part/systems modes can be beneficial. Schlumpf et al. (2019) demonstrated that trauma-focused treatment, based on the principles of Van der Hart et al. (2006), brings about desired changes in the neural networks involved in emotional control. It was shown that emotional over-regulation, manifesting as negative dissociative symptoms, was reduced.

Methods based on schema therapy can also be helpful (Huntjens et al., 2019; Jacob & Arntz, 2013; Young et al., 2003). Understanding the operation of schema modes in close relationships can support the process of building new patterns of intimacy and integrating the Healthy Adult mode. However, it is important to note that the use of schema therapy in individuals with emotional neglect experiences and dissociative personality structure may require adaptation and modification. A critical aspect here appears to be understanding the age at which individual schema modes are formed and whether they are based on a dissociative personality structure. It can be anticipated that, in the case of schema modes formed through traumatic dissociation, working with individual modes will require adapting methods to the cognitive and emotional capabilities typical of the age when each mode was formed. This approach is similar to the principles outlined by Van der Hart et al. (2006).

Finally, it is worth considering the possibility of psychotherapeutic work on emotional regulation disorders. We assume that individuals who have experienced emotional neglect may exhibit an increased threshold for recognising their emotions. This means that work on emotion regulation should include attempts to lower this threshold. Therapeutic methods based on mindfulness may be beneficial here (e.g., Cladder-Micus et al., 2023; Dumarkaite et al., 2021). Although studies on the effectiveness of mindfulness-based methods in the context of emotional trauma may raise methodological concerns (Zhang et al., 2021), the mindful observation of one's experiences, including somatic aspects, appears to be a very promising tool for expanding awareness of one's experiences.

Emotional education and experiential emotional processing are elements of many therapeutic approaches. However, given the repeatedly mentioned assumption that individuals emotionally neglected may experience personality fragmentation, therapeutic methods that consider closely tailored emotional contact in the therapist-patient relationship and provide significant attention to the patient's emotional needs deserve special attention. Therapy that enhances self-compassion facilitates the reduction of post-traumatic disorder symptoms (Winders et al., 2020). The metacognitive processing of beliefs about emotions, which is the focus of emotional schema therapy (Leahy, 2015), can help manage tension (e.g., Daneshmandi et al., 2014; Davoodi, 2014; Herbert & Forman, 2012; Leahy, 2007; Zorn et al., 2008).

Furthermore, transdiagnostic interventions aimed at increasing insights into emotionality, reducing discomfort avoidance, emotional self-regulation, and caring for individual needs should be particularly effective. Therapeutic methods that meet these needs are included in the Unified Protocol for transdiagnostic treatment of emotional disorders (Barlow et al., 2020). The usefulness of this method in individuals who have experienced trauma has been demonstrated (e.g., Hood et al., 2021; O'Donnell et al., 2021).

However, there is still a need for further research to fully understand and identify protective factors for individuals who have experienced emotional neglect in childhood. Due to time and length constraints we have necessarily left many potential leads for future exploration, as our main goal was to point out at least some of the contemporary problems of, and support mechanisms for, children experiencing emotional neglect so that their suffering could stop happening in silence.

References

A-Tjak, J. G. L., Morina, N., Boendermaker, W. J., Topper, M., & Emmelkamp, P. M. G. (2020). Explicit and implicit attachment and the outcomes of acceptance and commitment therapy and cognitive behavioral therapy for depression. *BMC Psychiatry, 20*(1), 155. https://doi.org/10.1186/s12888-020-02547-7

Abarca-Gómez, L., Abdeen, Z. A., Hamid, Z. A., Abu-Rmeileh, N. M., Acosta-Cazares, B., Acuin, C., ... & Ezzati, M. (2017). Worldwide trends in body-mass index, underweight, overweight, and obesity from 1975 to 2016: A pooled analysis of 2416 population-based measurement studies in 128.9 million children, adolescents, and adults. *The Lancet, 390*(10113), 2627–2642. https://doi.org/10.1016/S0140-6736(17)32129-3

Abels, M., Vanden Abeele, M., van Telgen, T., & van Meijl, H. (2018). Nod, nod, ignore: An exploratory observational study on the relation between parental mobile media use and parental responsiveness towards young children. In E. M. Luef & M. M. Marin (Eds.), *The talking species: Perspectives on the evolutionary, neuronal, and cultural foundations of language* (pp. 195–228). Uni-Press Verlag.

Abitante, G., Haraden, D. A., Pine, A., Cole, D., & Garber, J. (2022). Trajectories of positive and negative affect across adolescence: Maternal history of depression and adolescent sex as predictors. *Journal of Affective Disorders, 315*, 96–104.

Abu-Akel, A., & Shamay-Tsoory, S. (2011). Neuroanatomical and neurochemical bases of theory of mind. *Neuropsychologia, 49*(11), 2971–2984. https://doi.org/10.1016/j.neuropsychologia.2011.07.012

Acerbi, A. (2016). A cultural evolution approach to digital media. *Frontiers in Human Neuroscience, 10*, 636. https://doi.org/10.3389/fnhum.2016.00636

Ackerley, R., Backlund Wasling, H., Liljencrantz, J., Olausson, H., Johnson, R. D., & Wessberg, J. (2014). Human C-tactile afferents are tuned to the temperature of a skin-stroking caress. *The Journal of Neuroscience: The Official Journal of the Society for Neuroscience, 34*(8), 2879–2883. https://doi.org/10.1523/JNEUROSCI.2847-13.2014

Ainsworth, M. D. S., Blehar, M. C., Waters, E., & Wall, S. (2015). *Patterns of attachment: A psychological study of the strange situation.* Lawrence Erlbaum.

Alamiri, D. F., Arshad, H., Atif, F., Chauhan, S., Sohail, S., Safdar, M., ... & Anam, M. (2023). Emotional and psychological well-being in children with chronic medical conditions: A cross-sectional comparative study with healthy peers. *International Journal of Medical Science in Clinical Research and Review, 6*(06), 1043–1050. https://doi.org/10.5281/zenodo.10157205

Alexandre, G. C., Nadanovsky, P., Moraes, C. L., & Reichenheim, M. (2010). The presence of a stepfather and child physical abuse, as reported by a sample of Brazilian mothers in Rio de Janeiro. *Child Abuse & Neglect, 34*(12), 959–966. https://doi.org/10.1016/j.chiabu.2010.06.005

Algood, C. L., Hong, J. S., Gourdine, R. M., & Williams, A. B. (2011). Maltreatment of children with developmental disabilities: An ecological systems analysis. *Children and Youth Services Review, 33*(7), 1142–1148. https://doi.org/10.1016/j.childyouth.2011.02.003

Ali, E., Letourneau, N., & Benzies, K. (2021). Parent-child attachment: A principle-based concept analysis. *SAGE Open Nursing, 7*, 23779608211009000. https://doi.org/10.1177/23779608211009000

Alink, L. R. A., Mesman, J., van Zeijl, J., Stolk, M. N., Juffer, F., Koot, H. M. , … van IJzendoorn, M. H. (2006). The early childhood aggression curve: Development of physical aggression in 10-to 50-month-old children. *Child Development, 77*(4), 954–966. https://doi.org/10.1111/j.1467-8624.2006.00912.x

Allen, R. E., & Oliver, J. M. (1982). The effects of child maltreatment on language development. *Child Abuse & Neglect, 6*(3), 299–305. Retrieved from http://www.ncbi.nlm.nih.gov/pubmed/6892313

Allum, N., Patulny, R., Read, S., & Sturgis, P. (2010). Re-evaluating the links between social trust, institutional trust and civic association in Europe. In J. Stillwell (Ed.), *Understanding population trends and processes* (pp. 1–13). Springer. https://doi.org/10.1007/978-90-481-8750-8_13

Alter, B. J., Aung, M. S., Strigo, I. A., & Fields, H. L. (2020). Onset hyperalgesia and offset analgesia: Transient increases or decreases of noxious thermal stimulus intensity robustly modulate subsequent perceived pain intensity. *PloS One, 15*(12), e0231124. https://doi.org/10.1371/journal.pone.0231124

Althoff, M. L. (2023). The development of the mentalization ability. In: *Mentalizing power and powerlessness*. Springer. https://doi.org/10.1007/978-3-662-66119-2_2

Alutaybi, A., Al-Thani, D., McAlaney, J., & Ali, R. (2020). Combating fear of missing out (FoMO) on social media: The FoMO-R method. *International Journal of Environmental Research and Public Health, 17*(17), 6128. https://doi.org/10.3390/ijerph17176128

American Psychiatric Association, DSM-5 Task Force. (2013). *Diagnostic and statistical manual of mental disorders: DSM-5™* (5th ed.). American Psychiatric Publishing, Inc. https://doi.org/10.1176/appi.books.9780890425596

Anderson, D. R., & Hanson, K. G. (2017). Screen media and parent–child interactions. In R. Barr & D. N. Linebarger (Eds.), *Media exposure during infancy and early* childhood (pp. 173–194). Springer.

Ang, R. (2024). *Promoting children's mental health and wellbeing: Importance of partnerships in building resilient and empathic children*. Routledge.

Angelakis, I., Austin, J. L., & Gooding, P. (2020). Association of childhood maltreatment with suicide behaviors among young people: A systematic review and meta-analysis. *JAMA Network Open, 3*(8), https://doi.org/10.1001/jamanetworkopen.2020.12563

Antonovsky, A. (1979). *Health, stress, and coping*. San Francisco, CA: Jossey-Bass.

Arega, N. T. (2023). Mental health and psychosocial support interventions for children affected by armed conflict in low-and middle-income countries: A systematic review. *Child & Youth Care Forum*. https://doi.org/10.1007/s10566-023-09741-0

Atkinson, M., & Hornby, G. (2002). *Mental health handbook for schools*. Routledge Falmer.

Atzil, S., Touroutoglou, A., Rudy, T., Salcedo, S., Feldman, R., Hooker, J. M., ... & Barrett, L. F. (2017). Dopamine in the medial amygdala network mediates human bonding. *Proceedings of the National Academy of Sciences of the United States of America, 114*(9), 2361–2366. https://doi.org/10.1073/pnas.1612233114

Aust, S., Härtwig, E. A., Heuser, I., & Bajbouj, M. (2013). The role of early emotional neglect in alexithymia. *Psychological Trauma: Theory, Research, Practice, and Policy, 5*(3), 225–232. https://doi.org/10.1037/a0027314

Avdibegović, E., & Brkić, M. (2020). Child neglect - Causes and consequences. *Psychiatria Danubina, 32*(Suppl 3), 337–342.

Avila-Varela D. S., Arias-Trejo N., & Mani N. (2021). A longitudinal study of the role of vocabulary size in priming effects in early childhood. *Journal of Experimental Child Psychology, 205*, 105071. https://doi.org/10.1016/j.jecp.2020.105071

Baker, A. J. L. (2009). Adult recall of childhood psychological maltreatment: Definitional strategies and challenges. *Children and Youth Services Review, 31*(7), 703–714. https://doi.org/10.1016/j.childyouth.2009.03.001

Ban, J., & Oh, I. (2016). Mediating effects of teacher and peer relationships between parental abuse/neglect and emotional/behavioral problems. *Child Abuse and Neglect, 61*, 35–42. https://doi.org/10.1016/j.chiabu.2016.09.010

Barlow, D. H., Harris, B. A., Eustis, E. H., & Farchione, T. J. (2020). The unified protocol for transdiagnostic treatment of emotional disorders. *World Psychiatry, 19*(2), 245–246. https://doi.org/10.1002/wps.20748

Barr R, Lauricella A, Zack E, & Calvert SL (2010). Infant and early childhood exposure to adult-directed and child-directed television programming: Relations with cognitive skills at age four. *Merrill-Palmer Quarterly* (1982-), 21–48.

Barry, R. A., & Kochanska, G. (2010). A longitudinal investigation of the affective environment in families with young children: From infancy to early school age. *Emotion, 10*(2), 237–249. https://doi.org/10.1037/a0018485

Bauman, Z. (2009). Education in the liquid-modern setting. *Power and Education, 1*(2), 157–166. https://doi.org/10.2304/power.2009.1.2.157

Beck, J. S. (2011). *Cognitive therapy: Basics and beyond* (2nd ed.). Guilford Press.

Becker, M., Repantis, D., Dresler, M., & Kühn, S. (2022). Cognitive enhancement: Effects of methylphenidate, modafinil, and caffeine on latent memory and resting state functional connectivity in healthy adults. *Human Brain Mapping, 43*(14), 4225–4238. https://doi.org/10.1002/hbm.25949

Behrens, T. E., Hunt, L. T., Woolrich, M. W., & Rushworth, M. F. (2008). Associative learning of social value. *Nature, 456*(7219), 245–249. https://doi.org/10.1038/nature07538

Bennett, C., Melvin, G. A., Quek, J., Saeedi, N., Gordon, M. S., & Newman, L. K. (2019). Perceived invalidation in adolescent borderline personality disorder: An investigation of parallel reports of caregiver responses to negative emotions. *Child Psychiatry and Human Development, 50*(2), 209–221. https://doi.org/10.1007/s10578-018-0833-5

Bergen, D. (1998). Development of the sense of humor. In W. Ruch (Ed.), *The sense of humor: Explorations of a personality characteristic* (pp. 329–360). Mouton de Gruyter.

Bernath, M. S., & Feshbach, N. D. (1995). Children's trust: Theory, assessment, development, and research directions. *Applied and Preventive Psychology, 4*, 1–19.

Berndt, T. J. (2004). Children's friendships: Shifts over a half-century in perspectives on their development and their effects. *Merrill-Palmer Quarterly, 50*(3), 206–223. http://www.jstor.org/stable/23096162

Bernstein, M. J., & Claypool, H. M. (2012). Social exclusion and pain sensitivity: Why exclusion sometimes hurts and sometimes numbs. *Personality & social psychology bulletin, 38*(2), 185–196. https://doi.org/10.1177/0146167211422449

Beukeboom, C. J., & Pollmann, M. (2021). Partner phubbing: Why using your phone during interactions with your partner can be detrimental for your relationship. *Computers in Human Behavior, 124*, 106932. https://doi.org/10.1016/j.chb.2021.106932

Bickart, K. C., Hollenbeck, M. C., Barrett, L. F., & Dickerson, B. C. (2012). Intrinsic amygdala-cortical functional connectivity predicts social network size in humans. *The Journal of Neuroscience: The Official Journal of the Society for Neuroscience, 32*(42), 14729–14741. https://doi.org/10.1523/JNEUROSCI.1599-12.2012

Bickel, J., Bridgemohan, C., Sideridis, G., & Huntington, N. (2015). Child and family characteristics associated with age of diagnosis of an autism spectrum disorder in a tertiary care setting. *Journal of Developmental and Behavioral Pediatrics, 36*(1), 1–7. https://doi.org/10.1097/DBP.0000000000000117

Biringen, Z. (2000). Emotional availability: Conceptualization and research findings. *American Journal of Orthopsychiatry, 70*, 104–114. doi:10.1037/h0087711

Bogin, B. (2003). The human pattern of growth and development in paleontological perspective. In J. L. Thompson, G. E. Krovitz, & A. J. Nelson (Eds.), *Patterns of growth and development in the genus Homo* (pp. 15–44). Cambridge University Press.

Borgogna, N. C., McDermott, R. C., Aita, S. L., & Kridel, M. M. (2019). Anxiety and depression across gender and sexual minorities: Implications for transgender, gender nonconforming, pansexual, demisexual, asexual, queer, and questioning individuals. *Psychology of Sexual Orientation and Gender Diversity, 6*, 54–63. https://doi.org/10.1037/sgd0000306

Bornstein, M. H., Suwalsky, J. T., & Breakstone, D. A. (2012). Emotional relationships between mothers and infants: Knowns, unknowns, and unknown unknowns. *Development and Psychopathology, 24*(1), 113–123. https://doi.org/10.1017/S0954579411000708

Bosson, J. K., Brown, R. P., Zeigler-Hill, V., & Swann, W. B., Jr. (2003). Self-enhancement tendencies among people with high explicit self-esteem: The moderating role of implicit self-esteem. *Self and Identity, 2*(3), 169–187. https://doi.org/10.1080/15298860309029

Bostrom N. (2005). In defense of posthuman dignity. *Bioethics, 19*(3), 202–214. https://doi.org/10.1111/j.1467-8519.2005.00437.x

Bowlby, J. (1969). *Attachment and loss*, Vol. 1: Attachment. Attachment and Loss. Basic Books.

Boyd, D. G., & Bee, H. L. (2013). *The developing child* (13th ed.). Pearson Education Limited.

Bradbury, L. L., & Shaffer, A. (2012). Emotion dysregulation mediates the link between childhood emotional maltreatment and young adult romantic relationship satisfaction. *Journal of Aggression, Maltreatment & Trauma, 21*(6), 497–515. https://doi.org/10.1080/10926771.2012.678466

Brassard, M. R., & Donovan, K. L. (2006). Defining psychological maltreatment. In M. M. Freerick, J. F. Knutson, P. K. Trickett, & S. M. Flanzer (Eds.), *Child abuse and neglect: Definitions, classifications, & a framework for research* (pp. 151–197). Paul H. Brookes Publishing Co., Inc.

Braun, K., & Bock, J. (2011). The experience-dependent maturation of prefronto-limbic circuits and the origin of developmental psychopathology: Implications for the pathogenesis and therapy of behavioural disorders. *Developmental Medicine & Child Neurology, 53*(Suppl 4), 14–18. https://doi.org/10.1111/j.1469-8749.2011.04056.x

Braune-Krickau, K., Schneebeli, L., Pehlke-Milde, J., Gemperle, M., Koch, R., & von Wyl, A. (2021). Smartphones in the nursery: Parental smartphone use and parental sensitivity and responsiveness within parent-child interaction in early childhood (0–5 years): A scoping review. *Infant Mental Health Journal, 42*(2), 161–175. https://doi.org/10.1002/imhj.21908

Breen, A. V., Lewis, S. P., & Sutherland, O. (2013). Brief report: Non-suicidal self-injury in the context of self and identity development. *Journal of Adult Development*, 20, 57–62.

Briere, J., & Rickards, S. (2007). Self-awareness, affect regulation, and relatedness: Differential sequels of childhood versus adult victimization experiences. *Journal of Nervous and Mental Disease, 195*(6), 497–503. https://doi.org/10.1097/NMD.0b013e31803044e2

Brito, N. H., & Noble, K. G. (2014). Socioeconomic status and structural brain development. *Frontiers in Neuroscience, 8*, 276. https://doi.org/10.3389/fnins.2014.00276

Brontenbrenner, U. (1986). Ecology of the family as a context for human development: Research perspectives. *Developmental Psychology, 22*(6), 723–742.

Bronfenbrenner, U. (1989). Ecological systems theory. In R. Vasta (Ed.), *1989 Six Theories of Child Development: Revised Formulations and Current Issues* (Vol. 6). JAI Press, Greenwich, CT.

Brookman-Frazee, L., Stadnick, N., Chlebowski, C., Baker-Ericzén, M., & Ganger, W. (2018). Characterizing psychiatric comorbidity in children with autism spectrum disorder receiving publicly funded mental health services. *Autism: The International Journal of Research and Practice, 22*(8), 938–952. https://doi.org/10.1177/1362361317712650

Brothers, L. (2002). The social brain: A project for integrating primate behavior and neurophysiology in a new domain. In J. T. Cacioppo, G. G. Berntson, R. Adolphs, C. S. Carter, R. J. Davidson, M. McClintock, … & S. E. Taylor (Eds.), *Foundations in social neuroscience* (pp. 27–51). MIT Press. https://doi.org/10.7551/mitpress/3077.003.0029

Brown, D. (2023). Childhood experiences, growing up "in care," and trust: A quantitative analysis. *Children and Youth Services Review, 144*, 106734. https://doi.org/10.1016/j.childyouth.2022.106734

Brüne, M. (2016). *Textbook of evolutionary psychiatry & psychosomatic medicine. The origins of psychopathology* (2nd ed.). Oxford Press.

Burger C. (2022). Humor styles, bullying victimization and psychological school adjustment: Mediation, moderation and person-oriented analyses. *International Journal of Environmental Research and Public Health, 19*(18), 11415. https://doi.org/10.3390/ijerph191811415

Burgess Moser, M., Johnson, S. M., Dalgleish, T. L., Lafontaine, M. F., Wiebe, S. A., & Tasca, G. A. (2016). Changes in relationship-specific attachment in emotionally focused couple therapy. *Journal of Marital and Family Therapy, 42*(2), 231–245. https://doi.org/10.1111/jmft.12139

Burns, D. J., & Brady, J. (1992). A cross-cultural comparison of the need for uniqueness in Malaysia and the United States. *The Journal of Social Psychology, 132*(4), 487–495. https://doi.org/10.1080/00224545.1992.9924728

Busfield, J. (2010). 'A pill for every ill': Explaining the expansion in medicine use. *Social Science & Medicine, 70*(6), 934–941. doi: 10.1016/j.socscimed.2009.10.068. Epub 2010 Jan 22. PMID: 20096496.

Buss, D. (2015). *Evolutionary psychology: The new science of the mind* (5th ed.). Psychology Press.

Cacchioni, T., & Wolkowitz, C. (2011). Treating women's sexual difficulties: The body work of sexual therapy. *Sociology of Health & Illness, 33*(2), 266–279. https://doi.org/10.1111/j.1467-9566.2010.01288.x

Cai, H., Zou, X., Feng, Y., Liu, Y., & Jing, Y. (2018). Increasing need for uniqueness in contemporary China: Empirical evidence. *Frontiers in Psychology, 9*, 554. https://doi.org/10.3389/fpsyg.2018.00554

Cameron, G., Freymond, N., Cornfield, D., & Palmer, S. (2007). Positive possibilities for child and family welfare: Expanding the Anglo-American child protection paradigm. In G. Cameron, N. Coady, & G. R. Adams (Eds.), *Moving toward positive systems of child and family welfare: Current issues and future directions.* Wilfrid Laurier University Press.

Cann, A., & Collette, C. (2014). Sense of humor, stable affect, and psychological well-being. *Europe's Journal of Psychology, 10*(3), 464–479. https://doi.org/10.5964/ejop.v10i3.746

Cannon, W. B. (2016). *Bodily changes in pain, hunger, fear and rage: An account of recent researches into the function of emotional excitement.* Martino Fine Books.

Cao, H., Ma, R., Li, X., Liang, Y., Wu, Q., Chi, P., Li, J. B., & Zhou, N. (2022). Childhood emotional maltreatment and adulthood romantic relationship well-being: A multilevel, meta-analytic review. *Trauma, Violence, & Abuse, 23*(3), 778–794. https://doi.org/10.1177/1524838020975895

Caponnetto, P., Casu, M., Amato, M., Cocuzza, D., Galofaro, V., La Morella, A., ... & Vella, M. C. (2021). The effects of physical exercise on mental health: From cognitive improvements to risk of addiction. *International Journal of Environmental Research and Public Health, 18*(24), 13384. https://doi.org/10.3390/ijerph182413384

Carlson, E. B., Dalenberg, C., & McDade-Montez, E. (2012). Dissociation in posttraumatic stress disorder part 1: Definitions and review of research. *Psychological Trauma: Theory, Research, Practice, and Policy, 4*(5), 479–489. https://doi.org/10.1037/a0027748

Carmen, R. A., Guitar, A. E., & Dillon, H. M. (2012). Ultimate answers to proximate questions: The evolutionary motivations behind tattoos and body piercings in popular culture. *Review of General Psychology, 16*(2), 134–143. https://doi.org/10.1037/a0027908

Carr, L. J., Dunsiger, S. I., Lewis, B., Ciccolo, J. T., Hartman, S., Bock, B., Dominick, G., & Marcus, B. H. (2013). Randomized controlled trial testing an internet physical activity intervention for sedentary adults. *Health Psychology: Official Journal of the Division of Health Psychology, American Psychological Association, 32*(3), 328–336. https://doi.org/10.1037/a0028962

CASEL. (2022, March 11). *Fundamentals of SEL.* Retrieved April 30, 2024, from https://casel.org/fundamentals-of-sel/

Casey, B. J., Heller, A. S., Gee, D. G., & Cohen, A. O. (2019). Development of the emotional brain. *Neuroscience Letters, 693,* 29–34. https://doi.org/10.1016/j.neulet.2017.11.055

Caslini, M., Bartoli, F., Crocamo, C., Dakanalis, A., Clerici, M., & Carrà, G. (2016). Disentangling the association between child abuse and eating disorders: A systematic review and meta-analysis. *Psychosomatic Medicine, 78*(1), 79–90. https://doi.org/10.1097/PSY.0000000000000233

Cassels, M., van Harmelen, A. L., Neufeld, S., Goodyer, I., Jones, P. B., & Wilkinson, P. (2018). Poor family functioning mediates the link between childhood adversity and adolescent nonsuicidal self-injury. *Journal of Child Psychology and Psychiatry, and Allied Disciplines, 59*(8), 881–887. https://doi.org/10.1111/jcpp.12866

Čater, M., & Majdič, G. (2022). How early maternal deprivation changes the brain and behavior? *European Journal of Neuroscience, 55*(9), 2058–2075. https://doi.org/10.1111/ejn.15238

Chatton, M. A. (2017). *The experience of smartphone use amongst parents of 0–3-year olds.* Pro Quest LLC.

Chen, H. Z., & Xiao, W. (2014). An analysis of the Chinese parents' education-anxiety. *Journal of National Academy of Education Administration, 2,* 18–23.

Chester, D. S., Pond, R. S., Jr, Richman, S. B., & Dewall, C. N. (2012). The optimal calibration hypothesis: How life history modulates the brain's social pain network. *Frontiers in Evolutionary Neuroscience, 4,* 10. https://doi.org/10.3389/fnevo.2012.00010

Choe D. (2021). Longitudinal relationships amongst child neglect, social relationships, and school dropout risk for culturally and linguistically diverse adolescents. *Child Abuse & Neglect, 112,* 104891. https://doi.org/10.1016/j.chiabu.2020.104891

Christakis, D. A., Gilkerson, J., Richards, J. A., Zimmerman, F. J., Garrison, M. M., Xu, D., Gray, S., & Yapanel, U. (2009). Audible television and decreased adult words, infant vocalizations, and conversational turns: A population-based study. *Archives of Pediatrics & Adolescent Medicine, 163*(6), 554–558. https://doi.org/10.1001/archpediatrics.2009.61

Cicchetti, D., & Toth, S. L. (2005). Child maltreatment. *Annual Review of Clinical Psychology, 1,* 409–438. https://doi.org/10.1146/annurev.clinpsy.1.102803.144029

Cladder-Micus, M. B., Vrijsen, J. N., Fest, A., Spijker, J., Donders, A. R. T., Becker, E. S., & Speckens, A. E. M. (2023). Follow-up outcomes of mindfulness-based cognitive therapy (MBCT) for patients with chronic, treatment-resistant depression. *Journal of Affective Disorders, 335,* 410–417. https://doi.org/10.1016/j.jad.2023.05.023

Claes, L., Luyckx, K., & Bijttebier, P. (2014). Non-suicidal self-injury in adolescents: Prevalence and associations with identity formation above and beyond depression. *Personality and Individual Differences, 61–62,* 101–104. https://doi.org/10.1016/j.paid.2013.12.019

Clark, D. M., Ehlers, A., McManus, F., Hackmann, A., Fennell, M., Campbell, H., … & Louis, B. (2003). Cognitive therapy versus fluoxetine in generalized social phobia: A randomized placebo-controlled trial. *Journal of Consulting and Clinical Psychology, 71*(6), 1058–1067. https://doi.org/10.1037/0022-006X.71.6.1058

Clément, S., & Tereno, S. (2023). Attachment, feeding practices, family routines and childhood obesity: A systematic review of the literature. *International Journal of Environmental Research and Public Health, 20*(8), 5496. https://doi.org/10.3390/ijerph20085496

Cohen, J., McCabe, E. M., Michelli, N. M., & Pickeral, T. (2009). School climate: Research, policy, practice, and teacher education. *Teachers College Record, 111*(1), 180–213. https://doi.org/10.1177/016146810911100108

Collins, W. A. (Ed.). (1984). *Development during middle childhood: The years from six to twelve.* National Academy Press.

Collins, W. A., Welsh, D. P., & Furman, W. (2009). Adolescent romantic relationships. *Annual Review of Psychology, 60,* 631–652. https://doi.org/10.1146/annurev.psych.60.110707.163459

Colvert, E., Rutter, M., Beckett, C., Castle, J., Groothues, C., Hawkins, A., ... & Sonuga-Barke, E. J. (2008). Emotional difficulties in early adolescence following severe early deprivation: Findings from the English and Romanian adoptees study. *Development and Psychopathology, 20*(2), 547–567. https://doi.org/10.1017/S0954579408000278

Conrad, P. (2007). *The medicalization of society: On the transformation of human conditions into treatable disorders.* Johns Hopkins University Press

Cooper, R. J. (2006). The impact of child abuse on children's play: A conceptual model. *Occupational Therapy International, 13*(4), 249–263. https://doi.org/10.1002/oti.127

Cort, N. A., Toth, S. L., Cerulli, C., & Rogosch, F. (2011). Maternal intergenerational transmission of childhood multitype maltreatment. *Journal of Aggression, Maltreatment & Trauma, 20*(1), 20–39. https://doi.org/10.1080/10926771.2011.537740

Cosmides, L. (1989). The logic of social exchange: Has natural selection shaped how humans reason? Studies with the Wason selection task. *Cognition, 31*(3), 187–276. https://doi.org/10.1016/0010-0277(89)90023-1

Coveney, C., Gabe, J., & Williams, S. (2011). The sociology of cognitive enhancement: Medicalisation and beyond. *Health Sociology Review, 20*(4), 381–393. https://doi.org/10.5172/hesr.2011.20.4.381

Cowie, H. & Myers, C-A. (Eds.) (2018). *School bullying and mental health: Risks, intervention and prevention.* Routledge.

Coyne, S. M., Linder, J. R., Booth, M., Keenan-Kroff, S., Shawcroft, J. E., & Yang, C. (2021). Princess power: Longitudinal associations between engagement with princess culture in preschool and gender stereotypical behavior, body esteem, and hegemonic masculinity in early adolescence. *Child Development, 92*(6), 2413–2430. doi: 10.1111/cdev.13633. Epub 2021 Jul 20. PMID: 34287828.

Creech, S. K., & Misca, G. (2017). Parenting with PTSD: A review of research on the influence of PTSD on parent-child functioning in military and veteran families. *Frontiers in Psychology, 8,* 1101–1108. https://doi.org/10.3389/fpsyg.2017.01101

Crittenden, P. M. (1999). Atypical attachment in infancy and early childhood among children at developmental risk. VII. Danger and development: The organization of self-protective strategies. *Monographs of the Society for Research in Child*

Development, 64(3), 145–171; discussion 213–20. doi: 10.1111/1540-5834.00037. PMID: 10597546.

Culp, R. E., Watkins, R. V., Lawrence, H., Letts, D., Kelly, D. J., & Rice, M. L. (1991). Maltreated children's language and speech development: Abused, neglected, and abused and neglected. *First Language, 11*(33, Pt 3), 377–389. https://doi.org/10.1177/014272379101103305

Cycyk, L. M., & De Anda, S. (2021). Media exposure and language experience: Examining associations from home observations in Mexican immigrant families in the US. *Infant Behavior & Development, 63*, 101554. https://doi.org/10.1016/j.infbeh.2021.101554

Cycyk, L. M., & Hammer, C. S. (2020). Beliefs, values, and practices of Mexican immigrant families towards language and learning in toddlerhood: Setting the foundation for early childhood education. *Early Childhood Research Quarterly, 52*(Part A), 25–37. https://doi.org/10.1016/j.ecresq.2018.09.009

Czub, T. (2003). The importance of shame in the socialization process. In A. Brzezińska, S. Jabłoński, & M. Marchow (Eds.), *Invisible sources. Opportunities for development in childhood* (pp. 71–83). Fundacji Humaniora. [in Polish]

Dam, V. A. T., Dao, N. G., Nguyen, D. C., Vu, T. M. T., Boyer, L., Auquier, P., ... & Zhang, M. W. B. (2023). Quality of life and mental health of adolescents: Relationships with social media addiction, Fear of Missing out, and stress associated with neglect and negative reactions by online peers. *PloS One, 18*(6), e0286766. https://doi.org/10.1371/journal.pone.0286766

Damian, A. J., Oo, M., Bryant, D., & Gallo, J. J. (2021). Evaluating the association of adverse childhood experiences, mood and anxiety disorders, and suicidal ideation among behavioral health patients at a large federally qualified health center. *PLoS ONE, 16*(7), e0254385. https://doi.org/10.1371/journal.pone.0254385

Daneshmandi, S., Izadikhah, Z., Kazemi, H., & Mehrabi, H. (2014). The effectiveness of emotional schema therapy on emotional schemas of female victims of child abuse and neglect. *Journal of Shahid Sadoughi University of Medical Sciences, 22*(5), 1481–1494. http://jssu.ssu.ac.ir/article-1-2652-en.html

Dansby Olufowote, R. A., Fife, S. T., Schleiden, C., & Whiting, J. B. (2020). How can I become more secure?: A grounded theory of earning secure attachment. *Journal of Marital and Family Therapy, 46*(3), 489–506. https://doi.org/10.1111/jmft.12409

Daunic, A. P., Aydin, B., Corbett, N. L., Smith, S. W., Boss, D., & Crews, E. (2023). Social-emotional learning intervention for K–1 students at risk for emotional and behavioral disorders: Mediation effects of social-emotional learning on school adjustment. *Behavioral Disorders, 49*(1), 17–30. https://doi.org/10.1177/01987429231185098

Davies, C. A., Spence, J. C., Vandelanotte, C., Caperchione, C. M., & Mummery, W. K. (2012). Meta-analysis of internet-delivered interventions to increase physical activity levels. *The International Journal of Behavioral Nutrition and Physical Activity, 9*, 52. https://doi.org/10.1186/1479-5868-9-52

Davoodi, R. (2014). The effect of emotional schemas-based group therapy on emotion regulation in married women: A case study of Isfahan. *Advances in Environmental Biology, 8*(13), 1458–1465.

Dawson, D., Strodl, E., & Kitamura, H. (2022). Childhood maltreatment and disordered eating: The mediating role of emotion regulation. *Appetite, 172*, 105952. https://doi.org/10.1016/j.appet.2022.105952

De Graaf, J., Wann, D., & Naylor, T. H. (2005). *Affluenza: The all-consuming epidemic* (2nd ed.). Berrett-Koehler.

de Paúl, J., & Arruabarrena, M. I. (1995). Behavior problems in school-aged physically abused and neglected children in Spain. *Child Abuse & Neglect, 19*(4), 409–418. https://doi.org/10.1016/0145-2134(95)00009-W

Deen, B., & Saxe, R. (2019). Parts-based representations of perceived face movements in the superior temporal sulcus. *Human Brain Mapping, 40*(8), 2499–2510. https://doi.org/10.1002/hbm.24540

Del Giudice, M., Ellis, B. J., & Shirtcliff, E. A. (2011). The adaptive calibration model of stress responsivity. *Neuroscience and Biobehavioral Reviews, 35*(7), 1562–1592. https://doi.org/10.1016/j.neubiorev.2010.11.007

Demircioğlu, Z. I., & Göncü-Köse, A. (2023). Antecedents of problematic social media use and cyberbullying among adolescents: Attachment, the dark triad and rejection sensitivity. *Current Psychology, 42*, 31091–31109. https://doi.org/10.1007/s12144-022-04127-2

Deneault, A.-A., Hammond, S. I., & Madigan, S. (2023). A meta-analysis of child–parent attachment in early childhood and prosociality. *Developmental Psychology, 59*(2), 236–255. https://doi.org/10.1037/dev0001484

Dennis, T. A., & Kelemen, D. A. (2009). Preschool children's views on emotion regulation: Functional associations and implications for social-emotional adjustment. *International Journal of Behavioral Development, 33*(3), 243–252. https://doi.org/10.1177/0165025408098024

DeRosier, M. E., Kupersmidt, J. B., & Patterson, C. J. (1994). Children's academic and behavioral adjustment as a function of the chronicity and proximity of peer rejection. *Child Development, 65*(6), 1799–1813. https://doi.org/10.1111/j.1467-8624.1994.tb00850.x

DeWall, C. N., & Baumeister, R. F. (2006). Alone but feeling no pain: Effects of social exclusion on physical pain tolerance and pain threshold, affective forecasting, and interpersonal empathy. *Journal of Personality and Social Psychology, 91*(1), 1–15. https://doi.org/10.1037/0022-3514.91.1.1

Di Giunta, L., Lunetti, C., Gliozzo, G., Rothenberg, W. A., Lansford, J. E., Eisenberg, N., ... & Virzì, A. T. (2022). Negative parenting, adolescents' emotion regulation, self-efficacy in emotion regulation, and psychological adjustment. *International Journal of Environmental Research and Public Health, 19*(4), 2251. https://doi.org/10.3390/ijerph19042251

Di Giunta, L., Pastorelli, C., Thartori, E., Bombi, A. S., Baumgartner, E., Fabes, R. A., Martin, C. L., & Enders, C. K. (2018). Trajectories of Italian children's peer rejection: Associations with aggression, prosocial behavior, physical attractiveness, and adolescent adjustment. *Journal of Abnormal Child Psychology, 46*(5), 1021–1035. https://doi.org/10.1007/s10802-017-0373-7

Diamond, G., Diamond, G. M., & Levy, S. (2021). Attachment-based family therapy: Theory, clinical model, outcomes, and process research. *Journal of Affective Disorders, 294*, 286–295. https://doi.org/10.1016/j.jad.2021.07.005

Diener, E., Lucas, R. E., & Scollon, C. N. (2006). Beyond the hedonic treadmill: Revising the adaptation theory of well-being. *The American Psychologist, 61*(4), 305–314. https://doi.org/10.1037/0003-066X.61.4.305

DiLillo, D., Peugh, J., Walsh, K., Panuzio, J., Trask, E., & Evans, S. (2009). Child maltreatment history among newlywed couples: A longitudinal study of marital outcomes and mediating pathways. *Journal of Consulting and Clinical Psychology, 77*(4), 680–692. https://doi.org/10.1037/a0015708

Dodge, K. A., Lansford, J. E., Burks, V. S., Bates, J. E., Pettit, G. S., Fontaine, R., & Price, J. M. (2003). Peer rejection and social information-processing factors in the development of aggressive behavior problems in children. *Child Development, 74*(2), 374–393. doi: 10.1111/1467-8624.7402004. PMID: 12705561; PMCID: PMC2764280.

Dollberg, D. G., & Hanetz-Gamliel, K. (2023). Therapeutic work to enhance parental mentalizing for parents with ACEs to support their children's mental health: A theoretical and clinical review. *Frontiers in Child and Adolescent Psychiatry, 2,* 1094206. https://doi.org/10.3389/frcha.2023.1094206

Domke, A.-K., Hartling, C., Stippl, A., Carstens, L., Gruzman, R., Bajbouj, M., Gärtner, M., & Grimm, S. (2023). The influence of childhood emotional maltreatment on cognitive symptoms, rumination, and hopelessness in adulthood depression. *Clinical Psychology & Psychotherapy, 30*(5), 1170–1178. https://doi.org/10.1002/cpp.2872

Dong, M., Anda, R. F., Felitti, V. J., Dube, S. R., Williamson, D. F., Thompson, T. J., Loo, C. M., & Giles, W. H. (2004). The interrelatedness of multiple forms of childhood abuse, neglect, and household dysfunction. *Child Abuse & Neglect, 28*(7), 771–784. https://doi.org/10.1016/j.chiabu.2004.01.008

Dong, S., Dong, Q., Chen, H., & Yang, S. (2022). Childhood emotional neglect and adolescent depression: The role of self-compassion and friendship quality. *Current Psychology.* https://doi.org/10.1007/s12144-022-03539-4

Dorahy, M. J., Middleton, W., Seager, L., Williams, M., & Chambers, R. (2016). Child abuse and neglect in complex dissociative disorder, abuse-related chronic PTSD, and mixed psychiatric samples. *Journal of Trauma & Dissociation, 17*(2), 223–236. https://doi.org/10.1080/15299732.2015.1077916

Dube, S. R., Felitti, V. J., Dong, M., & others. (2003). Childhood abuse, neglect, and household dysfunction and the risk of illicit drug use: The adverse childhood experiences study. *Pediatrics, 111*(3), 564. https://doi.org/10.1542/peds.111.3.564

Dubowitz, H., Black, M., Starr, R. H., & Zuravin, S. (1993). A conceptual definition of child neglect. *Criminal Justice and Behavior, 20*(1), 8–26. https://doi.org/10.1177/0093854893020001003

Dubowitz, H., Pitts, S. C., & Black, M. M. (2004). Measurement of three major subtypes of child neglect. *Child Maltreatment, 9*(4), 344–356. https://doi.org/10.1177/1077559504269191

Dumarkaite, A., Truskauskaite-Kuneviciene, I., Andersson, G., Mingaudaite, J., & Kazlauskas, E. (2021). Effects of mindfulness-based internet intervention on ICD-11 posttraumatic stress disorder and complex posttraumatic stress disorder symptoms: A pilot randomized controlled trial. *Mindfulness, 12*(11), 2754–2766. https://doi.org/10.1007/s12671-021-01739-w

Dunbar R. I. (2010). The social role of touch in humans and primates: Behavioural function and neurobiological mechanisms. *Neuroscience and Biobehavioral Reviews, 34*(2), 260–268. https://doi.org/10.1016/j.neubiorev.2008.07.001

Dunbar, R. I. M. (2022). Virtual touch and the human social world. *Current Opinion in Behavioral Sciences, 43,* 14–19. https://doi.org/10.1016/j.cobeha.2021.06.009

Dunbar, R. I., & Schultz, S. (2007). Evolution in the social brain. *Science, 317*(5843), 1344–1347. https://doi.org/10.1126/science.1145463

Dunn, M.G., Tarter, R.E., Mezzich, A.C., Vanyukov, M., Kirisci, L., & Kirillova, G. (2002). Origins and consequences of child neglect in substance abuse families. *Clinical Psychology Review, 22*, 1063–1090.

Duong, J., & Bradshaw, C. P. (2017). Links between contexts and middle to late childhood social-emotional development. *American Journal of Community Psychology, 60*(3–4), 538–554. https://doi.org/10.1002/ajcp.12201

Durlak, J. A., Weissberg, R. P., Dymnicki, A. B., Taylor, R. D., & Schellinger, K. B. (2011). The impact of enhancing students' social and emotional learning: A meta-analysis of school-based universal interventions. *Child Development, 82*, 405–432. https://doi.org/10.1111/j.1467-8624.2010.01564.x

Dziura, S. L., & Thompson, J. C. (2014). Social-network complexity in humans is associated with the neural response to social information. *Psychological Science, 25*(11), 2095–2101. https://doi.org/10.1177/0956797614549209

Eisenberg, N. (2020). Findings, issues, and new directions for research on emotion socialization. *Developmental Psychology, 56*(3), 664–670. https://doi.org/10.1037/dev0000906

Eisenberger, N. I. (2012). The neural bases of social pain: Evidence for shared representations with physical pain. *Psychosomatic Medicine, 74*(2), 126–135. https://doi.org/10.1097/PSY.0b013e3182464dd1

Eisenberger, N. I., & Lieberman, M. D. (2004). Why rejection hurts: A common neural alarm system for physical and social pain. *Trends in Cognitive Sciences, 8*(7), 294–300. https://doi.org/10.1016/j.tics.2004.05.010

Eisenberger, N. I., Jarcho, J. M., Lieberman, M. D., & Naliboff, B. D. (2006). An experimental study of shared sensitivity to physical pain and social rejection. *Pain, 126*(1), 132–138. https://doi.org/10.1016/j.pain.2006.06.024

Eisenberger, N. I., Lieberman, M. D., & Williams, K. D. (2003). Does rejection hurt? An FMRI study of social exclusion. *Science, 302*(5643), 290–292. https://doi.org/10.1126/science.1089134

Elias, L. J., & Abdus-Saboor, I. (2022). Bridging skin, brain, and behavior to understand pleasurable social touch. *Current Opinion in Neurobiology, 73*, 102527. https://doi.org/10.1016/j.conb.2022.102527

Elias, L. J., Succi, I. K., Schaffler, M. D., Foster, W., Gradwell, M. A., Bohic, M., ... & Abdus-Saboor, I. (2023). Touch neurons underlying dopaminergic pleasurable touch and sexual receptivity. *Cell, 186*(3), 577–590.e16. https://doi.org/10.1016/j.cell.2022.12.034

Elias, M. J., Zins, J. E., Weissberg, R. P., Frey, K. S., Greenberg, M. T., Haynes, N. M., & Shriver, T. P. (1997). *Promoting social and emotional learning: Guidelines for educators.* Association for Supervision and Curriculum Development.

Elias, N., Lemish, D., Dalyot, S., & Floegel, D. (2020). "Where are you?" An observational exploration of parental technoference in public places in the US and Israel. *Journal of Children and Media, 15*(3), 376–388. https://doi.org/10.1080/17482798.2020.1815228

Elliott, R., & Macdonald, J. (2021). Relational dialogue in emotion-focused therapy. *Journal of Clinical Psychology, 77*(2), 414–428. https://doi.org/10.1002/jclp.23069

Elzy, M. B. (2013). Emotional invalidation: An investigation into its definition, measurement, and effects. *USF Tampa Graduate Theses and Dissertations.* https://digitalcommons.usf.edu/etd/4670

Emde, R. N., & Easterbrooks, M. A. (1985). Assessing emotional availability in early development. InW. K. Frankenburg, R. N. Emde, &J. W. Sullivan (Eds.), *Early identification of children at risk. Topics in developmental psychobiology.* Springer. https://doi.org/10.1007/978-1-4899-0536-9_5

Endevelt-Shapira, Y., & Feldman, R. (2023). Mother–infant brain-to-brain synchrony patterns reflect caregiving profiles. *Biology, 12*(2), 284. https://doi.org/10.3390/biology12020284

Epkins, C. C., & Heckler, D. R. (2011). Integrating etiological models of social anxiety and depression in youth: Evidence for a cumulative interpersonal risk model. *Clinical Child and Family Psychology Review, 14*(4), 329–376. https://doi.org/10.1007/s10567-011-0101-8

Erickson, M. F., & Egeland, B. (2002). Child neglect. In J. E. B. Myers, L. Berliner, J. Briere, C. T. Hendrix, C. Jenny, & T. A. Reid (Eds.), *APSAC handbook on child maltreatment* (2nd ed., pp. 3–20). Sage Publications.

Erikson, E. H. (1968). *Identity: Youth and crisis.* Norton.

Ewing, E. S., Diamond, G., & Levy, S. (2015). Attachment-based family therapy for depressed and suicidal adolescents: Theory, clinical model and empirical support. *Attachment & Human Development, 17*(2), 136–156. https://doi.org/10.1080/14616734.2015.1006384

Fabris, M. A., Marengo, D., Longobardi, C., & Settanni, M. (2020). Investigating the links between fear of missing out, social media addiction, and emotional symptoms in adolescence: The role of stress associated with neglect and negative reactions on social media. *Addictive Behaviors, 106*, 106364. https://doi.org/10.1016/j.addbeh.2020.106364

Fassbinder, E., Schweiger, U., Martius, D., Brand-de Wilde, O., & Arntz, A. (2016). Emotion regulation in schema therapy and dialectical behavior therapy. *Frontiers in Psychology, 7*, 1373. https://doi.org/10.3389/fpsyg.2016.01373

Feldman, R. (2007). Parent–infant synchrony: Biological foundations and developmental outcomes. *Current Directions in Psychological Science, 16*(6), 340–345. https://doi.org/10.1111/j.1467-8721.2007.00532.x

Feldman, R., Rosenthal, Z., & Eidelman, A. I. (2014). Maternal-preterm skin-to-skin contact enhances child physiologic organization and cognitive control across the first 10 years of life. *Biological Psychiatry, 75*(1), 56–64. https://doi.org/10.1016/j.biopsych.2013.08.012

Felitti, V. J., Anda, R. F., Nordenberg, D., Williamson, D. F., Spitz, A. M., Edwards, V., Koss, M. P., & Marks, J. S. (1998). Relationship of childhood abuse and household dysfunction to many of the leading causes of death in adults. The Adverse Childhood Experiences (ACE) Study. *American Journal of Preventive Medicine, 14*(4), 245–258. https://doi.org/10.1016/s0749-3797(98)00017-8

Feng, M., & Zhou, G. (2023). Children's peer rejection trajectories and Internet gaming addiction: A five-wave growth mixture model. *International Journal of Behavioral Development, 47*(5), 375–383. https://doi.org/10.1177/01650254231182966

Fenning, R. M., Baker, B. L., & Juvonen, J. (2011). Emotion discourse, social cognition, and social skills in children with and without developmental delays. *Child Development, 82*(2), 717–731. http://www.jstor.org/stable/29782862

Fields-Olivieri, M. A., Cole, P. M., & Roben, C. K. P. (2020). Toddler emotion expressions and emotional traits: Associations with parent-toddler verbal conversation.

Infant Behavior & Development, 61, 101474. https://doi.org/10.1016/j.infbeh.2020.101474

Finzi, R., Har-Even, D., & Weizman, A. (2003). Comparison of ego defenses among physically abused children, neglected, and non-maltreated children. *Comprehensive Psychiatry, 44*(5), 388–395. https://doi.org/10.1016/S0010-440X(03)00106-8

Fitch, A., Lieberman, A. M., Luyster, R. J., & Arunachalam, S. (2020). Toddlers' word learning through overhearing: Others' attention matters. *Journal of Experimental Child Psychology, 193*, 104793. https://doi.org/10.1016/j.jecp.2019.104793

Flick, U. (2011). *Managing quality in qualitative research*. SAGE Publications, Ltd.

Fogel, A., Nwokah, E., Dedo, J. Y., Messinger, D., Dickson, K. L., Matusov, E., & Holt, S. A. (1992). Social process theory of emotion: A dynamic systems approach. *Social Development, 1*, 122–142. https://doi.org/10.1111/j.1467-9507.1992.tb00116.x

Foote, B., & Van Orden, K. (2016). Adapting dialectical behavior therapy for the treatment of dissociative identity disorder. *American Journal of Psychotherapy, 70*(4), 343–364. https://doi.org/10.1176/appi.psychotherapy.2016.70.4.343

Franco, A. de F., Mendonça, F. W., & Tuleski, S. C. (2020). Medicalização da infância: avanço ou retrocesso. *Nuances: Estudos Sobre Educação, 31*, 38–59. https://doi.org/10.32930/nuances.v31iesp.1.8289

Franz, L., Angold, A., Copeland, W., Costello, E. J., Towe-Goodman, N., & Egger, H. (2013). Preschool anxiety disorders in pediatric primary care: Prevalence and comorbidity. *Journal of the American Academy of Child and Adolescent Psychiatry, 52*(12), 1294–1303.e1. https://doi.org/10.1016/j.jaac.2013.09.008

Franz, M. R., Kumar, S. A., Brock, R. L., Calvi, J. L., & DiLillo, D. (2022). Parenting behaviors of mothers with posttraumatic stress: The roles of cortisol reactivity and negative emotion. *Journal of Family Psychology: Journal of the Division of Family Psychology of the American Psychological Association (Division 43), 36*(1), 130–139. https://doi.org/10.1037/fam0000865

Frewen, P., McPhail, I., Schnyder, U., Oe, M., & Olff, M. (2021). Global Psychotrauma Screen (GPS): psychometric properties in two internet-based studies. *European Journal of Psychotraumatology, 12*(1), 1–13. 10.1080/20008198.2021.1881725

Frith, U., & Frith, C. (2001). The biological basis of social interaction. *Current Directions in Psychological Science, 10*(5), 151–155. https://doi.org/10.1111/1467-8721.00137

Fukuyama, F. (1995). Social capital and the global economy. *Foreign Affairs, 74*(5), 89–103. https://doi.org/10.2307/20047302

Gajdzica, Z., Byra, S., Kołodziej-Zaleska, A., Rutkowska, K., & Dzienniak-Pulina, D. (2024). *Mental health and quality of life of adolescents with physical, intellectual and developmental disabilities*. Routledge.

Gaur, D. S., Jacka, B. P., Green, T. C., Samuels, E. A., Hadland, S. E., Krieger, M. S., Yedinak, J. L., & Marshall, B. D. L. (2020). US drug overdose mortality: 2009–2018 increases affect young people who use drugs. *The International Journal on Drug Policy, 85*, 102906. https://doi.org/10.1016/j.drugpo.2020.102906

Gazzaniga, M. (2008). *Human: The science behind what makes your brain unique*. Ecco.

Gear, R. W., Aley, K. O., & Levine, J. D. (1999). Pain-induced analgesia mediated by mesolimbic reward circuits. *The Journal of Neuroscience: The Official Journal of the Society for Neuroscience, 19*(16), 7175–7181. https://doi.org/10.1523/JNEUROSCI.19-16-07175.1999

Gibson, L. C. (2019). *Recovering from emotionally immature parents: Practical tools to establish boundaries and reclaim your emotional autonomy.* New Harbinger.

Giddens, A. (2006). *Sociology* (5th ed.). Polity Press.

Gigerenzer, G., & Garcia-Retamero, R. (2017). Cassandra's regret: The psychology of not wanting to know. *Psychological Review, 124*(2), 179–196. https://doi.org/10.1037/rev0000055

Gilbert P. (1997). The evolution of social attractiveness and its role in shame, humiliation, guilt and therapy. *The British Journal of Medical Psychology, 70 (Pt 2),* 113–147. https://doi.org/10.1111/j.2044-8341.1997.tb01893.x

Gilbert, P. (2000). Social mentalities: Internal 'social' conflicts and the role of inner warmth and compassion in cognitive therapy. In P. Gilbert & K. G. Bailey (Eds.), *Genes on the Couch: Explorations in evolutionary psychotherapy* (pp. unknown). Psychology Press.

Gilbert, R., Spatz Widom, C., Browne, K., Fergusson, D., Webb, E., & Janson, S. (2009). Burden and consequences of child maltreatment in high-income countries. *The Lancet, 373,* 68–81. https://doi.org/10.1016/S0140-6736(08)61706-7

Ginsburg, K. R. (2007). The importance of play in promoting healthy child development and maintaining strong parent-child bonds. *Pediatrics, 119*(1), 182–191. https://doi.org/10.1542/peds.2006-2697

Giotakos O. (2020). Neurobiology of emotional trauma. *Psychiatrike = Psychiatriki, 31*(2), 162–171. https://doi.org/10.22365/jpsych.2020.312.162

Glaser D. (2002). Emotional abuse and neglect (psychological maltreatment): A conceptual framework. *Child Abuse & Neglect, 26*(6–7), 697–714. https://doi.org/10.1016/s0145-2134(02)00342-3

Glaser, D. (2011). How to deal with emotional abuse and neglect: Further development of a conceptual framework (FRAMEA). *Child Abuse & Neglect, 35*(10), 866–875. https://doi.org/10.1016/j.chiabu.2011.08.002

Glickman, E. A., Choi, K. W., Lussier, A. A., Smith, B. J., & Dunn, E. C. (2021). Childhood emotional neglect and adolescent depression: Assessing the protective role of peer social support in a longitudinal birth cohort. *Frontiers in Psychiatry, 12,* 681176. https://doi.org/10.3389/fpsyt.2021.681176 Gobin, R. L., & Freyd, J. J. (2014). The impact of betrayal trauma on the tendency to trust. *Psychological Trauma: Theory, Research, Practice, and Policy, 6*(5), 505–511. https://doi.org/10.1037/a0032452

Gonzalez-Liencres, C., Shamay-Tsoory, S. G., & Brüne, M. (2013). Towards a neuroscience of empathy: Ontogeny, phylogeny, brain mechanisms, context and psychopathology. *Neuroscience and Biobehavioral Reviews, 37*(8), 1537–1548. https://doi.org/10.1016/j.neubiorev.2013.05.001

Goode, J. A., Fomby, P., Mollborn, S., & Limburg, A. (2019). Children's technology time in two US cohorts. *Child Indicators Research, 12*(3), 1107–1132. https://doi.org/10.1007/s12187-019-09675-x

Gordon-Hacker, A., & Gueron-Sela, N. (2020). Maternal use of media to regulate child distress: A double-edged sword? Longitudinal links to toddlers' negative emotionality. *Cyberpsychology, Behavior, and Social Networking, 23*(6), 400–405. https://doi.org/10.1089/cyber.2019.0487

Gordon, I., & Feldman, R. (2008). Synchrony in the triad: A microlevel process model of coparenting and parent-child interactions. *Family Process, 47*(4), 465–479. https://doi.org/10.1111/j.1545-5300.2008.00266.x

Gori, A., Topino, E., & Griffiths, M. D. (2023). The associations between attachment, self-esteem, fear of missing out, daily time expenditure, and problematic social media use: A path analysis model. *Addictive Behaviors, 141*, 107633. https://doi.org/10.1016/j.addbeh.2023.107633

Greenfield, P. M., Keller, H., Fuligni, A., & Maynard, A. (2003). Cultural pathways through universal development. *Annual Review of Psychology, 54*, 461–490. https://doi.org/10.1146/annurev.psych.54.101601.145221

Greenwald, A. G., & Banaji, M. R. (1995). Implicit social cognition: Attitudes, self-esteem, and stereotypes. *Psychological Review, 102*(1), 4–27. https://doi.org/10.1037/0033-295x.102.1.4

Griffith A. K. (2022). Parental burnout and child maltreatment during the COVID-19 pandemic. *Journal of Family Violence, 37*(5), 725–731. https://doi.org/10.1007/s10896-020-00172-2

Griffiths, R. R., Johnson, M. W., Richards, W. A., Richards, B. D., McCann, U., & Jesse, R. (2011). Psilocybin occasioned mystical-type experiences: Immediate and persisting dose-related effects. *Psychopharmacology (Berl), 218*(4), 649–665. doi: 10.1007/s00213-011-2358-5. Epub 2011 Jun 15. PMID: 21674151; PMCID: PMC 3308357.

Grill, J. D., & Coghill, R. C. (2002). Transient analgesia evoked by noxious stimulus offset. *Journal of Neurophysiology, 87*(4), 2205–2208. https://doi.org/10.1152/jn.00730.2001

Grummitt, L. R., Kelly, E. V., Barrett, E. L., Lawler, S., Prior, K. Stapinski, L. A., & Newton, N. C. (2022). Associations of childhood emotional and physical neglect with mental health and substance use in young adults. *Australian & New Zealand Journal of Psychiatry, 56*(4), 365–375. https://doi.org/10.1177/00048674211025691

Grzadzinski, R., Amso, D., Landa, R., Watson, L., Guralnick, M., Zwaigenbaum, L., ... & Piven, J. (2021). Pre-symptomatic intervention for autism spectrum disorder (ASD): Defining a research agenda. *Journal of Neurodevelopmental Disorders, 13*(1), 49. https://doi.org/10.1186/s11689-021-09393-y

Gupta, A., Kashyap, A., & Sidana, A. (2019). Dialectical behavior therapy in emotion dysregulation - Report of two cases. *Indian Journal of Psychological Medicine, 41*(6), 578–581. https://doi.org/10.4103/IJPSYM.IJPSYM_352_19

Guthrie, W., Swineford, L. B., Nottke, C., & Wetherby, A. M. (2013). Early diagnosis of autism spectrum disorder: Stability and change in clinical diagnosis and symptom presentation. *Journal of Child Psychology and Psychiatry, and Allied Disciplines, 54*(5), 582–590. https://doi.org/10.1111/jcpp.12008

Hampton, W. H., Unger, A., Von Der Heide, R. J., & Olson, I. R. (2016). Neural connections foster social connections: A diffusion-weighted imaging study of social networks. *Social Cognitive and Affective Neuroscience, 11*(5), 721–727. https://doi.org/10.1093/scan/nsv153

Hamre, B. K., & Pianta, R. C. (2001). Early teacher-child relationships and the trajectory of children's school outcomes through eighth grade. *Child Development, 72*(2), 625–638. http://www.jstor.org/stable/1132418

Hamre, B. K., & Pianta, R. C. (2005). Can instructional and emotional support in the first-grade classroom make a difference for children at risk of school failure? *Child Development, 76*(5), 949–967. https://doi.org/10.1111/j.1467-8624.2005.00889.x

Han, M., Jiang, G., Luo, H., & Shao, Y. (2021). Neurobiological bases of social networks. *Frontiers in Psychology, 12*, 626337. https://doi.org/10.3389/fpsyg.2021.626337

Hanakawa, T., Immisch, I., Toma, K., Dimyan, M. A., Van Gelderen, P., & Hallett, M. (2003). Functional properties of brain areas associated with motor execution and imagery. *Journal of Neurophysiology, 89*(2), 989–1002. https://doi.org/10.1152/jn.00132.2002

Handley, E. D., Russotti, J., Warmingham, J. M., Rogosch, F. A., Todd Manly, J., & Cicchetti, D. (2021). Patterns of child maltreatment and the development of conflictual emerging adult romantic relationships: An examination of mechanisms and gender moderation. *Child Maltreatment, 26*(4), 387–397. https://doi.org/10.1177/10775595211022837

Handlin, L., Novembre, G., Lindholm, H., Kämpe, R., Paul, E., & Morrison, I. (2023). Human endogenous oxytocin and its neural correlates show adaptive responses to social touch based on recent social context. *eLife, 12*, e81197. https://doi.org/10.7554/eLife.81197

Hanson, J. L., Nacewicz, B. M., Sutterer, M. J., Cayo, A. A., Schaefer, S. M., Rudolph, K. D., ... & Davidson, R. J. (2015). Behavioral problems after early life stress: Contributions of the hippocampus and amygdala. *Biological Psychiatry, 77*(4), 314–323. https://doi.org/10.1016/j.biopsych.2014.04.020

Harrington, S., Pascual-Leone, A., Paivio, S., Edmondstone, C., & Baher, T. (2021). Depth of experiencing and therapeutic alliance: What predicts outcome for whom in emotion-focused therapy for trauma? *Psychology and Psychotherapy, 94*(4), 895–914. https://doi.org/10.1111/papt.12342

Hayashi, M. (2022). Child psychological/emotional abuse and neglect: A definitional conceptual framework. *Journal of Child & Adolescent Trauma, 15*(4), 999–1010. https://doi.org/10.1007/s40653-022-00448-3

Head Zauche, L., Thul, T. A., Mahoney, A. E. D., & Stapel-Wax, J. L. (2016). Influence of language nutrition on children's language and cognitive development: An integrated review. *Early Childhood Research Quarterly, 36*(3), 318–333. https://doi.org/10.1016/j.ecresq.2016.01.015

Heim, C., Shugart, M., Craighead, W. E., & Nemeroff, C. B. (2010). Neurobiological and psychiatric consequences of child abuse and neglect. *Developmental Psychobiology, 52*(7), 671–690. https://doi.org/10.1002/dev.20494

Henden, E. (2023). Addiction and autonomy: Why emotional dysregulation in addiction impairs autonomy and why it matters. *Frontiers in Psychology, 14*, 1081810. https://doi.org/10.3389/fpsyg.2023.1081810

Herbert, J. D., & Forman, E. M. (2012). Emotional schema therapy: A bridge over troubled waters. In R. L. Leahy (Ed.), *Acceptance and mindfulness in cognitive behavior therapy: Understanding and applying the new therapies* (pp. 157–182). Wiley.

Hertenstein, M. J., & Campos, J. J. (2001). Emotion regulation via maternal touch. *Infancy, 2*(4), 549–566. https://doi.org/10.1207/S15327078IN0204_09

Hildyard, K. L., & Wolfe, D. A. (2002). Child neglect: Developmental issues and outcomes. *Child Abuse & Neglect, 26*(6–7), 679–695. https://doi.org/10.1016/S0145-2134(02)00341-1

Hindman, A. H., Farrow, J. M., Anderson, K., Wasik, B. A., & Snyder, P. A. (2021). Understanding child-directed speech around book reading in toddler classrooms: Evidence from early head start programs. *Frontiers in Psychology, 12*, 719783. https://doi.org/10.3389/fpsyg.2021.719783

Hipwell, A. E., Tung, I., Northrup, J., & Keenan, K. (2019). Transgenerational associations between maternal childhood stress exposure and profiles of infant emotional reactivity. *Development and Psychopathology, 31*(3), 887–898. https://doi.org/10.1017/S0954579419000324

Hochschild, A. R. (1983). *The managed heart: Commercialization of human feeling.* University of California Press.

Hoferichter, F., Kulakow, S., & Hufenbach, M. C. (2021). Support from parents, peers, and teachers is differently associated with middle school students' well-being. *Frontiers in Psychology, 12*, 758226. https://doi.org/10.3389/fpsyg.2021.758226

Hoffman, M. L. (2008). Empathy and prosocial behavior. In M. Lewis, J. M. Haviland-Jones, & L. F. Barrett (Eds.), *Handbook of emotions* (3rd ed., pp. 440–455). Guilford Publications.

Hoffmann, J. P. (2020). Academic underachievement and delinquent behavior. *Youth & Society, 52*(5), 728–755. https://doi.org/10.1177/0044118X18767035

Holodynski, M. (2009). Milestones and mechanisms of emotional development. In H. J. Markowitsch & B. Röttger-Rössler (Eds.), *Emotions as bio-cultural processes* (pp. 1–25). Springer.

Hong, J. S., & Espelage, D. L. (2012). A review of research on bullying and peer victimization in school: An ecological system analysis. *Aggression and Violent Behavior, 17*, 311–322. https://doi.org/10.1016/j.avb.2012.03.003

Hood, C. O., Southward, M. W., Bugher, C., & Sauer-Zavala, S. (2021). A preliminary evaluation of the Unified Protocol among trauma-exposed adults with and without PTSD. *International Journal of Environmental Research and Public Health, 18*(21), 11729. https://doi.org/10.3390/ijerph182111729

Hou, S., Twayigira, M., Luo, X., Song, L., Cui, X., Xie, Q., Shen, Y., Yang, F., & Yuan, X. (2023). The relationship between emotional neglect and non-suicidal self-injury among middle school students in China: The mediating role of social anxiety symptoms and insomnia. *BMC Psychiatry, 23*(1), 248. https://doi.org/10.1186/s12888-023-04735-7

Howe, D. (2005). *Child abuse and neglect: Attachment, development and intervention.* Palgrave Macmillan.

Howes, O. D., Rogdaki, M., Findon, J. L., Wichers, R. H., Charman, T., King, B. H., … & Murphy, D. G. (2018). Autism spectrum disorder: Consensus guidelines on assessment, treatment and research from the British Association for Psychopharmacology. *Journal of Psychopharmacology (Oxford, England), 32*(1), 3–29. https://doi.org/10.1177/0269881117741766

Hrdy, S. B. (2000). *Mother nature: Maternal instincts and how they shape the human species* (1st Ballantine Books ed.). Ballantine Books.

Huang, Y., Li, R., Fang, L., Wu, S., Wan, Y., He, H., Peng, C., & Wang, X. (2022). Relationship between family rearing style and 3–6 year old children's emotional and behavioral problems. *Chinese Journal of School Health,* (12), 242–246.

Hughes, C., & Ensor, R. (2006). Behavioural problems in 2-year-olds: Links with individual differences in theory of mind, executive function and harsh parenting. *Journal of Child Psychology and Psychiatry, and Allied Disciplines, 47*(5), 488–497. https://doi.org/10.1111/j.1469-7610.2005.01519.x

Hughes, J. (2004). *Citizen cyborg. Why democratic societies must respond to the redesigned human of the future.* West View Press, Perseus Books Group.

Huntjens, R. J. C., Rijkeboer, M. M., & Arntz, A. (2019). Schema therapy for dissociative identity disorder (DID): Rationale and study protocol. *European Journal of Psychotraumatology, 10*(1), 1571377. https://doi.org/10.1080/20008198.2019.1571377

Huot, R. L., Ladd, C. O., & Plotsky, P. M. (2007). Maternal deprivation. In G. Fink (Ed.), *Encyclopedia of stress* (2nd ed., pp. 667–674). Academic Press. https://doi.org/10.1016/B978-012373947-6.00250-6

Igarashi, H., Kikuchi, H., Kano, R., Mitoma, H., Shono, M., Hasui, C., & Kitamura, T. (2009). The inventory of personality organisation: Its psychometric properties among student and clinical populations in Japan. *Annals of General Psychiatry, 8*, 9. https://doi.org/10.1186/1744-859X-8-9

Ikeda, Y., Nishimura, Y., & Higuchi, S. (2019). Effects of the differences in mental states on the mirror system activities when observing hand actions. *Journal of Physiological Anthropology, 38*(1). https://doi.org/10.1186/s40101-018-0192-8

Infurna, M. R., Reichl, C., Parzer, P., Schimmenti, A., Bifulco, A., & Kaess, M. (2016). Associations between depression and specific childhood experiences of abuse and neglect: A meta-analysis. *Journal of Affective Disorders, 190*, 47–55. https://doi.org/10.1016/j.jad.2015.09.006

Insel, T. R., Gingrich, B. S., & Young, L. J. (2001). Oxytocin: Who needs it? *Progress in Brain Research, 133*, 59–66. https://doi.org/10.1016/s0079-6123(01)33005-4

Invitto, S., & Grasso, A. (2019). Chemosensory perception: A review on electrophysiological methods in "cognitive neuro-olfactometry." *Chemosensors, 7*(3), 45. https://doi.org/10.3390/chemosensors7030045

Isenhardt, A., Kamenowski, M., Manzoni, P., Haymoz, S., Jacot, C., & Baier, D. (2021). Identity diffusion and extremist attitudes in adolescence. *Frontiers in Psychology, 12*, 711466. https://doi.org/10.3389/fpsyg.2021.711466

Jacob, G. A., & Arntz, A. (2013). Schema therapy for personality disorders: A review. *International Journal of Cognitive Therapy, 6*, 171–185. https://doi.org/10.1521/ijct.2013.6.2.171

James, O. (2007). *Affluenza: How to be successful and stay sane.* Vermilion.

Jańczak M. O. (2023). Mentalization, emotional dysregulation and attachment to alternative attachment figures in retrospectively defined earned secure adults. *Current Issues in Personality Psychology, 12*(1), 30–40. https://doi.org/10.5114/cipp/172328

Jankowiak, B. (2019). Young people in crisis – The experience of being neglected among adolescents as a neglected area of theory and research. *Nauki o Wychowaniu. Studia Interdyscyplinarne, 8*(2), 73–86. [in Polish]

Järbrink, K., & Knapp, M. (2001). The economic impact of autism in Britain. *Autism: The International Journal of Research and Practice, 5*(1), 7–22. https://doi.org/10.1177/1362361301005001002

Jauch, M., Rudert, S. C., & Greifeneder, R. (2022). Social pain by non-social agents: Exclusion hurts and provokes punishment even if the excluding source is a computer. *Acta Psychologica, 230*, 103753. https://doi.org/10.1016/j.actpsy.2022.103753

Jessar, A. J., Hamilton, J. L., Flynn, M., Abramson, L. Y., & Alloy, L. B. (2017). Emotional clarity as a mechanism linking emotional neglect and depressive symptoms during early adolescence. *The Journal of Early Adolescence, 37*(3), 414–432. https://doi.org/10.1177/0272431615609157

Jewkes, R. K., Dunkle, K., Nduna, M., Jama, P. N., & Puren, A. (2010). Associations between childhood adversity and depression, substance abuse and HIV and HSV2 incident infections in rural South African youth. *Child Abuse & Neglect, 34*(11), 833–841. https://doi.org/10.1016/j.chiabu.2010.05.002

Jia, Y., Way, N., Ling, G., Yoshikawa, H., Chen, X., Hughes, D., Ke, X., & Lu, Z. (2009). The influence of student perceptions of school climate on socio-emotional and academic adjustment: A comparison of Chinese and American adolescents. *Child Development, 80*(5), 1514–1530. https://doi.org/10.1111/j.1467-8624.2009.01348.x

Jin, X., Xu, B., Lin, H., Chen, J., Xu, R., & Jin, H. (2023). The influence of childhood emotional neglect on emotional face processing in young adults. *Acta Psychologica, 232*, 103814. https://doi.org/10.1016/j.actpsy.2022.103814

Johnson, K. V., & Dunbar, R. I. (2016). Pain tolerance predicts human social network size. *Scientific Reports, 6*, 25267. https://doi.org/10.1038/srep25267

Johnson, S. M., & Whiffen, V. E. (1999). Made to measure: Adapting emotionally focused couple therapy to partners' attachment styles. *Clinical Psychology: Science and Practice, 6*(4), 366–381. https://doi.org/10.1093/clipsy.6.4.366

Jones, P. W., Thornton, A. E., Jones, A. A., Knerich, V. M., Lang, D. J., Woodward, M. L., ... & Gicas, K. M. (2020). Amygdala nuclei volumes are selectively associated with social network size in homeless and precariously housed persons. *Frontiers in Behavioral Neuroscience, 14*, 97. https://doi.org/10.3389/fnbeh.2020.00097

Jones, S., Martin, R., & Pilbeam, D. (1992). *The Cambridge encyclopedia of human evolution*. Cambridge University Press.

Jordan, C. H., & Zeigler-Hill, V. (2013). The perils and pitfalls of (some) high self-esteem. In V. Zeigler-Hill (Ed.), *Self-esteem* (pp. 80–98). Psychology Press.

Juul, S. H., Hendrix, C., Robinson, B., Stowe, Z. N., Newport, D. J., Brennan, P. A., & Johnson, K. C. (2015). Maternal early-life trauma and affective parenting style: The mediating role of HPA-axis function. *Archives of Women's Mental Health, 1*, 1–7. https://doi.org/10.1007/s00737-015-0528-x

Kabali, H. K., Irigoyen, M. M., Nunez-Davis, R., Budacki, J. G., Mohanty, S. H., Leister, K. P., & Bonner, R. L., Jr (2015). Exposure and use of mobile media devices by young children. *Pediatrics, 136*(6), 1044–1050. https://doi.org/10.1542/peds.2015-2151

Kajanoja, J., Karukivi, M., Scheinin, N. M., Ahrnberg, H., Karlsson, L., & Karlsson, H. (2021). Early-life adversities and adult attachment in depression and alexithymia. *Development and Psychopathology, 33*(4), 1428–1436. https://doi.org/10.1017/S0954579420000607

Kalinichev, M., & Francis, D. (2010). Maternal deprivation. In *Encyclopedia of behavioral neuroscience* (pp. 173–177). Elsevier. https://doi.org/10.1016/B978-0-08-045396-5.00017-8

Kantor, G. K., Holt, M. K., Mebert, C. J., Straus, M. A., Drach, K. M., Ricci, L. R., Macallum, C. A., & Brown, W. (2004). Development and preliminary psychometric properties of the multidimensional neglectful behavior scale-child report. *Child Maltreatment, 9*, 409–428.

Karelas G. D. (2011). Social marketing self-esteem: A socio-medical approach to high-risk and skin tone alteration activities. *International Journal of Dermatology, 50*(5), 590–592. https://doi.org/10.1111/j.1365-4632.2011.05010.x

Karim, F., Oyewande, A. A., Abdalla, L. F., Chaudhry Ehsanullah, R., & Khan, S. (2020). Social media use and its connection to mental health: A systematic review. *Cureus, 12*(6), e8627. https://doi.org/10.7759/cureus.8627

Kauffman, J. M. & Badar, J. (eds) (2023). *Navigating students' mental health in the wake of Covid 19: Using public health crises to inform research and practice.* Routledge.

Kaufman Kantor, G., Holt, M. K., Mebert, C. J., Straus, M. A., Drach, K. M., Ricci, L. R., MacAllum, C. A., & Brown, W. (2004). Development and psychometric properties of the Child Self-Report Multidimensional Neglectful Behavior Scale (MNBS-CR). *Child Maltreatment, 9*(4), 409–429. https://doi.org/10.1177/1077559504269192

Kazarian, S. S., Moghnie, L., & Martin, R. A. (2010). Perceived parental warmth and rejection in childhood as predictors of humor styles and subjective happiness. *Europe's Journal of Psychology, 6*(3), 71–93. https://doi.org/10.5964/ejop.v6i3.209

Ke, H., Vuong, Q. C., & Geangu, E. (2022). Three- and six-year-old children are sensitive to natural body expressions of emotion: An event-related potential emotional priming study. *Journal of Experimental Child Psychology, 224*, Article 105497. https://doi.org/10.1016/j.jecp.2022.105497

Kelleher, K., Chaffin, M., Hollenberg, J., & Fischer, E. (1994). Alcohol and drug disorders among physically abusive and neglectful parents in a community-based sample. *American Journal of Public Health, 84*(10), 1586–1590. https://doi.org/10.2105/ajph.84.10.1586

Kendall-Tackett, K. A., & Eckenrode, J. (1996). The effects of neglect on academic achievement and disciplinary problems: A developmental perspective. *Child Abuse & Neglect, 20*(3), 161–169. https://doi.org/10.1016/s0145-2134(95)00139-5

Keverne, E. B., Martensz, N. D., & Tuite, B. (1989). Beta-endorphin concentrations in cerebrospinal fluid of monkeys are influenced by grooming relationships. *Psychoneuroendocrinology, 14*(1–2), 155–161. https://doi.org/10.1016/0306-4530(89)90065-6

Keyes, K. M., Eaton, N. R., Krueger, R. F., McLaughlin, K. A., Wall, M. M., Grant, B. F., & Hasin, D. S. (2012). Childhood maltreatment and the structure of common psychiatric disorders. *British Journal of Psychiatry, 200*(2), 107–115. https://doi.org/10.1192/bjp.bp.111.093062

Khourochvili, M. (2017). Technology and caregiver-child interaction: The effects of parental mobile device use on infants (Doctoral dissertation). York University, Toronto. Retrieved from https://yorkspace.library.yorku.ca/xmlui/handle/10315/34309

Kidd, L., & Rowland, C. F. (2021). The effect of language-focused professional development on the knowledge and behaviour of preschool practitioners. *Journal of Early Childhood Literacy, 21*(1), 27–59. https://doi.org/10.1177/1468798418803664

Kildare, C. A., & Middlemiss, W. (2017). Impact of parents mobile device use on parent-child interaction: A literature review. *Computers in Human Behavior, 75*, 579–593. https://doi.org/10.1016/j.chb.2017.06.003

Kim, B.-R., Chow, S.-M., Bray, B., & Teti, D. M. (2017). Trajectories of mothers' emotional availability: Relations with infant temperament in predicting attachment security. *Attachment & Human Development, 19*(1), 38–57. https://doi.org/10.1080/14616734.2016.1252780

Kim, J., & Cicchetti, D. (2010). Longitudinal pathways linking child maltreatment, emotion regulation, peer relations, and psychopathology. *Journal of Child Psychology and Psychiatry, and Allied Disciplines, 51*(6), 706–716. https://doi.org/10.1111/j.1469-7610.2009.02202.x

Kininmonth, A. R., Smith, A., Carnell, S., Steinsbekk, S., Fildes, A., & Llewellyn, C. (2021). The association between childhood adiposity and appetite assessed using the child eating behavior questionnaire and Baby eating behavior questionnaire: A systematic review and meta-analysis. *Obesity Reviews, 22*(5), e13169. https://doi.org/10.1111/obr.13169

Kirby, L. A., Moraczewski, D., Warnell, K., Velnoskey, K., & Redcay, E. (2018). Social network size relates to developmental neural sensitivity to biological motion. *Developmental Cognitive Neuroscience, 30*, 169–177. https://doi.org/10.1016/j.dcn.2018.02.012

Klein, D., & Kuiper, N. (2006). Humor styles, peer relationships, and bullying in middle childhood. *HUMOR, 19*(4), 383–404. https://doi.org/10.1515/HUMOR.2006.019

Klika, J. B., Haboush-Deloye, A., & Linkenbach, J. (2019). Hidden protections: Identifying social norms associated with child abuse, sexual abuse, and neglect. *Child and Adolescent Social Work Journal, 36*, 5–14. https://doi.org/10.1007/s10560-018-0595-8

Koenig, A. L., Cicchetti, D., & Rogosch, F. A. (2000). Child compliance/noncompliance and maternal contributors to internalization in maltreating and nonmaltreating dyads. *Child Development, 71*, 1018–1032. doi:10.1111/1467-8624.00206

Kopp, C. B. (1989). Regulation of distress and negative emotions: A developmental view. *Developmental Psychology, 25*(3), 343–354. https://doi.org/10.1037/0012-1649.25.3.343

Kourkouta, L., & Papathanassiou, I. V. (2014). Communication in nursing practice. *Materia Socio-medica, 26*(1), 65–67. DOI: 10.5455/msm.2014.26.65-67

Krause-Utz, A., Frost, R., Winter, D., & Elzinga, B. M. (2017). Dissociation and alterations in brain function and structure: Implications for borderline personality disorder. *Current Psychiatry Reports, 19*(1), 6. https://doi.org/10.1007/s11920-017-0757-y

Kumari, V. (2020). Emotional abuse and neglect: time to focus on prevention and mental health consequences. *British Journal of Psychiatry, 217*(5), 597–599. doi: 10.1192/bjp.2020.154. PMID: 32892766; PMCID: PMC7589986.

Kupersmidt, J. B., & Coie, J. D. (1990). Preadolescent peer status, aggression, and school adjustment as predictors of externalizing problems in adolescence. *Child Development, 61*(5), 1350–1362. https://doi.org/10.1111/j.1467-8624.1990.tb02866.x

Kwak, S., Joo, W. T., Youm, Y., & Chey, J. (2018). Social brain volume is associated with in-degree social network size among older adults. *Proceedings. Biological Sciences, 285*(1871), 20172708. https://doi.org/10.1098/rspb.2017.2708

Lambie, J. A., & Lindberg, A. (2016). The role of maternal emotional validation and invalidation on children's emotional awareness. *Merrill-Palmer Quarterly, 62*(2), 129–157. https://doi.org/10.13110/merrpalmquar1982.62.2.0129

Lamm, C., Batson, C. D., & Decety, J. (2007). The neural substrate of human empathy: Effects of perspective-taking and cognitive appraisal. *Journal of Cognitive Neuroscience, 19*(1), 42–58. https://doi.org/10.1162/jocn.2007.19.1.42

Lanius, R. A. (2015). Trauma-related dissociation and altered states of consciousness: A call for clinical, treatment, and neuroscience research. *European Journal of Psychotraumatology, 6*(1), 27905. https://doi.org/10.3402/ejpt.v6.27905

LaParo K. M., Hamre B. K., Locasale-Crouch J., Pianta R. C., Bryant D., Early D., ... & Burchinal, M. (2009). Quality in kindergarten classrooms: Observational evidence for the need to increase children's learning opportunities in early education classrooms. *Early Education and Development, 20*, 657–692. https://doi.org/10.1080/10409280802541965

Lavigne, H. J., Hanson, K. G., & Anderson, D. R. (2015). The influence of television coviewing on parent language directed at toddlers. *Journal of Applied Developmental Psychology, 36*, 1–10. https://doi.org/10.1016/j.appdev.2014.11.004

Lawrence, P. J., Murayama, K., & Creswell, C. (2019). Systematic review and meta-analysis: Anxiety and depressive disorders in offspring of parents with anxiety disorders. *Journal of the American Academy of Child and Adolescent Psychiatry, 58*(1), 46–60. https://doi.org/10.1016/j.jaac.2018.07.898

Lawson, D. M., & Quinn, J. (2013). Complex trauma in children and adolescents: Evidence-based practice in clinical settings. *Journal of Clinical Psychology, 69*(5), 497–509. https://doi.org/10.1002/jclp.21990

Leaf, J. B., Cihon, J. H., Leaf, R., McEachin, J., Liu, N., Russell, N., ... & Khosrowshahi, D. (2022). Concerns about ABA-based intervention: An evaluation and recommendations. *Journal of Autism and Developmental Disorders, 52*(6), 2838–2853. https://doi.org/10.1007/s10803-021-05137-y

Leahy, R. L. (2007). Emotional schemas and resistance to change in anxiety disorders. *Cognitive and Behavioral Practice, 14*(1), 36–45. https://doi.org/10.1016/j.cbpra.2006.08.001

Leahy, R. L. (2015). *Emotional schema therapy.* Guilford Press.

Leclère, C., Viaux, S., Rabain, D., Khun-Franck, L., Dubois, C., Camon-Senechal, L., ... & Missonnier, S. (2018). Video feedback in situations of emotional neglect: A tool for assessment and care of early interactions? *Annales Médico-psychologiques, revue psychiatrique, 176*(3), 296–300. https://doi.org/10.1016/j.amp.2018.01.003

Lee, J. K., Johnson, E. G., & Ghetti, S. (2017). Hippocampal development: Structure, function and implications. In D. Hannula & M. Duff (Eds.), *The Hippocampus from cells to systems* (pp. 47–70). Springer. https://doi.org/10.1007/978-3-319-50406-3_6

Lee, S. W., Bae, G. Y., Rim, H. D., Lee, S. J., Chang, S. M., Kim, B. S., & Won, S. (2018). Mediating effect of resilience on the association between emotional neglect and depressive symptoms. *Psychiatry Investigation, 15*(1), 62–69. https://doi.org/10.4306/pi.2018.15.1.62

Lench, H. C., Flores, S. A., & Bench, S. W. (2011). Discrete emotions predict changes in cognition, judgment, experience, behavior, and physiology: A meta-analysis of experimental emotion elicitations. *Psychological Bulletin, 137*(5), 834–855. https://doi.org/10.1037/a0024244

Leschak, C. J. & Eisenberger, N. I. (2018). The role of social relationships in the link between olfactory dysfunction and mortality. *PLoS ONE, 13*(5), e0196708. https://doi.org/10.1371/journal.pone.0196708

Lester, B. M., Conradt, E., LaGasse, L. L., Tronick, E. Z., Padbury, J. F., & Marsit, C. J. (2018). Epigenetic programming by maternal behavior in the human infant. *Pediatrics, 142*(4), e20171890. https://doi.org/10.1542/peds.2017-1890

Levine, L. E., Waite, B. M., Bowman, L. L., & Kachinsky, K. (2019). Mobile media use by infants and toddlers. *Computers in Human Behavior, 94*, 92–99. https://doi.org/10.1016/j.chb.2018.12.045

Li, S., Lin, Y., Liu, P., & Xing, S. (2023). Childhood emotional neglect and adolescent depression: Roles of maladaptive self-cognition and friendship quality. *Children and Youth Services Review, 155*, 107272.

Lilleston, P. S., Goldmann, L., Verma, R. K., & McCleary-Sills, J. (2017). Understanding social norms and violence in childhood: Theoretical underpinnings and strategies for intervention. *Psychology, Health & Medicine, 22*, 122–134. https://doi.org/10.1080/13548506.2016.1271954

Lindenfors, P., Wartel, A., & Lind, J. (2021). 'Dunbar's number' deconstructed. *Biology Letters, 17*(5), 20210158. https://doi.org/10.1098/rsbl.2021.0158

Linebarger DL, & Vaala SE (2010). Screen media and language development in infants and toddlers: An ecological perspective. *Developmental Review, 30*(2), 176–202.

Lipari, R. N., & Van Horn, S. L. (2017). Children living with parents who have a substance use disorder. In *The CBHSQ report* (pp. 1–7). Substance Abuse and Mental Health Services Administration (US).

Liu, Y., Li, S., Lin, W., Li, W., Yan, X., Wang, X., Pan, X., Rutledge, R. B., & Ma, Y. (2019). Oxytocin modulates social value representations in the amygdala. *Nature Neuroscience, 22*(4), 633–641. https://doi.org/10.1038/s41593-019-0351-1

Löken, L. S., Wessberg, J., Morrison, I., McGlone, F., & Olausson, H. (2009). Coding of pleasant touch by unmyelinated afferents in humans. *Nature Neuroscience, 12*(5), 547–548. https://doi.org/10.1038/nn.2312

Longobardi, E., Spataro, P., Putnick, D. L., & Bornstein, M. H. (2016). Noun and verb production in maternal and child language: Continuity, stability, and prediction across the second year of life. *Language Learning and Development: The Official Journal of the Society for Language Development, 12*(2), 183–198. https://doi.org/10.1080/15475441.2015.1048339

López-López, J. A., Kwong, A. S. F., Washbrook, L., Tilling, K., Fazel, M. S., & Pearson, R. M. (2021). Depressive symptoms and academic achievement in UK adolescents: A cross-lagged analysis with genetic covariates. *Journal of Affective Disorders, 284*, 104–113. https://doi.org/10.1016/j.jad.2021.01.091

Lorber, M. F., & O'Leary, S. G. (2005). Mediated paths to overreactive discipline: Mothers' experienced emotion, appraisals, and physiological responses. *Journal of Consulting and Clinical Psychology, 73*(5), 972–981. https://doi.org/10.1037/0022-006X.73.5.972

Ludwig, S., & Rostain, A. (2009). Family function and dysfunction. In W. B. Carey, A. C. Crocker, W. L. Coleman, E. R. Elias, & H. M. Feldman (Eds.), *Developmental-behavioral pediatrics* (4th ed., pp. 103-118). W.B. Saunders. https://doi.org/10.1016/B978-1-4160-3370-7.00010-9

Lumley, M. A., Neely, L. C., & Burger, A. J. (2007). The assessment of alexithymia in medical settings: Implications for understanding and treating health problems. *Journal of Personality Assessment, 89*, 230–246. https://doi.org/10.1080/00223890701629698

Luna, B., & Wright, C. (2016). Adolescent brain development: Implications for the juvenile criminal justice system. In *APA handbook of psychology and juvenile justice* (pp. 91–116). American Psychological Association. https://doi.org/10.1037/14643-005

Lyons, R. M., Yule, A. M., Schiff, D., Bagley, S. M., & Wilens, T. E. (2019). Risk factors for drug overdose in young people: A systematic review of the literature. *Journal of Child and Adolescent Psychopharmacology, 29*(7), 487–497. https://doi.org/10.1089/cap.2019.0013

Lyvers, M., Mayer, K., Needham, K., & Thorberg, F. A. (2019). Parental bonding, adult attachment, and theory of mind: A developmental model of alexithymia and alcohol-related risk. *Journal of Clinical Psychology, 75*(7), 1288–1304. https://doi.org/10.1002/jclp.22772

Ma, C., & Song, J. (2023). Parental emotional neglect and academic procrastination: The mediating role of future self-continuity and ego depletion. *PeerJ, 11*, e16274. https://doi.org/10.7717/peerj.16274

MacDonald, G., & Leary, M. R. (2005). Why does social exclusion hurt? The relationship between social and physical pain. *Psychological Bulletin, 131*(2), 202–223. https://doi.org/10.1037/0033-2909.131.2.202

Machin, A. J., & Dunbar, R. I. M. (2011). The brain opioid theory of social attachment: A review of the evidence. *Behaviour, 148*(9/10), 985–1025. http://www.jstor.org/stable/23034206

Macht, M. (2008). How emotions affect eating: A five-way model. *Appetite, 50*(1), 1–11. https://doi.org/10.1016/j.appet.2007.07.002

Mack, A. H. (2012). Infant media exposure and toddler development. *Yearbook of Psychiatry and Applied Mental Health, 2012*, 22–23. https://doi.org/10.1016/j.ypsy.2011.09.025

Maguire, L. K., Niens, U., McCann, M., & Connolly, P. (2016). Emotional development among early school-age children: Gender differences in the role of problem behaviours. *Educational Psychology, 36*(8), 1408–1428. https://doi.org/10.1080/01443410.2015.1034090

Maguire, S. A., Williams, B., Naughton, A. M., Cowley, L. E., Tempest, V., Mann, M. K., Teague, M., & Kemp, A. M. (2015). A systematic review of the emotional, behavioural and cognitive features exhibited by school-aged children experiencing neglect or emotional abuse. *Child: Care, Health and Development, 41*(5), 641–653. https://doi.org/10.1111/cch.12227

Mahfoud, D., Pardini, S., Mróz, M., Hallit, S., Obeid, S., Akel, M., Novara, C., & Brytek-Matera, A. (2023). Profiling orthorexia nervosa in young adults: The role of obsessive behaviour, perfectionism, and self-esteem. *Journal of Eating Disorders, 11*(1), 188. https://doi.org/10.1186/s40337-023-00915-8

Majorano, M., Musetti, A., Brondino, M., & Corsano, P. (2015). Loneliness, emotional autonomy, and motivation for solitary behavior during adolescence. *Journal of Child and Family Studies, 24*(11), 3436–3447. https://doi.org/10.1007/s10826-015-0145-3

Malafouris, L. (2010). The brain–artefact interface (BAI): A challenge for archaeology and cultural neuroscience. *Social Cognitive and Affective Neuroscience, 5*(2–3), 264–273. https://doi.org/10.1093/scan/nsp057

Manly, J. T., Lynch, M., Oshri, A., Herzog, M., & Wortel, S. N. (2013). The impact of neglect on initial adaptation to school. *Child Maltreatment, 18*(3), 155–170. https://doi.org/10.1177/1077559513496144

Marcia, J. E. (1966). Development and validation of ego-identity status. *Journal of Personality and Social Psychology, 3*(5), 551–558. https://doi.org/10.1037/h0023281

Marcoen, A., Goossens, L., & Caes, P. (1987). Loneliness in pre-through late adolescence: Exploring the contributions of a multidimensional approach. *Journal of Youth and Adolescence, 16*, 561–577. https://doi.org/10.1007/BF02138821

Marryat, L., Thompson, L., Minnis, H., & Wilson, P. (2014). Associations between social isolation, pro-social behaviour and emotional development in preschool aged children: A population based survey of kindergarten staff. *BMC Psychology, 2*, 44. https://doi.org/10.1186/s40359-014-0044-1

Marsh, H., & Kleitman, S. (2002). Extracurricular school activities: The good, the bad, and the nonlinear. *Harvard Educational Review, 72*(4), 464–515. https://doi.org/10.17763/haer.72.4.051388703v7v7736

Marshall, B., Cardon, P., Poddar, A., & Fontenot, R. (2013). Does sample size matter in qualitative research?: A review of qualitative interviews in is research. *Journal of Computer Information Systems, 54*(1), 11–22. https://doi.org/10.1080/088744 17.2013.11645667

Martin, R. A., Puhlik-Doris, P., Larsen, G., Gray, J., & Weir, K. (2003). Individual differences in the uses of humor and their relation to psychological well-being: Development of the Humor Styles Questionnaire. *Journal of Research in Personality, 37*(1), 48–75. https://doi.org/10.1016/S0092-6566(02)00534-2

Martin, S., & Strodl, E. (2023). The relationship between childhood trauma, eating behaviours, and the mediating role of metacognitive beliefs. *Appetite, 188*, 106975. https://doi.org/10.1016/j.appet.2023.106975

Matejczuk, J. (2014). *Child development: Preschool age: age 2/3–5/6 years.* Educational Research Institute. [in Polish]

Mathews, B., Pacella, R., Dunne, M. P., Simunovic, M., & Marston, C. (2020). Improving measurement of child abuse and neglect: A systematic review and analysis of national prevalence studies. *PLOS ONE, 15*(1), e0227884. https://doi.org/10.1371/journal.pone.0227884

McClure, P. K. (2017). Tinkering with technology and religion in the digital age: The effects of Internet use on religious belief, behavior, and belonging. *Journal for the Scientific Study of Religion, 56*(3), 481–497. http://www.jstor.org/stable/26651880

McCormick, M. P., Cappella, E., O'Connor, E. E., & McClowry, S. G. (2015). Context matters for social-emotional learning: Examining variation in program impact by dimensions of school climate. *American Journal of Community Psychology, 56*(1–2), 101–119. https://doi.org/10.1007/s10464-015-9733-z

McGhee, P. E. (2010). *Humor: The lighter path to resilience and health.* AuthorHouse.

McWhirter, B. T. (1990). Loneliness: A review of current literature, with implications for counseling and research. *Journal of Counseling & Development, 68*(4), 417–422. https://doi.org/10.1002/j.1556-6676.1990.tb02521.x

Meins, E., Fernyhough, C., Wainwright, R., Das Gupta, M., Fradley, E., & Tuckey, M. (2002). Maternal mind–mindedness and attachment security as predictors of theory of mind understanding. *Child Development, 73*(6), 1715–1726. https://doi.org/10.1111/1467-8624.00501

Mendelsohn, A. L., Brockmeyer, C. A., Dreyer, B. P., Fierman, A. H., Berkule-Silberman, S. B., & Tomopoulos, S. (2010). Do verbal interactions with infants during electronic media exposure mitigate adverse impacts on their language development as toddlers? *Infant and Child Development, 19*(6), 577–593. https://doi.org/10.1002/icd.711

Merriam, S. B. (2009). *Qualitative research: A guide to design and implementation* (3rd ed., p. 46). Jossey-Bass.

Mikolajczak, M., & Luminet, O. (2006). Is alexithymia affected by situational stress or is it a stable trait related to emotion regulation? *Personality and Individual Differences, 40*(7), 1399–1408. https://doi.org/10.1016/j.paid.2005.10.020

Mikolajczak, M., Gross, J. J., & Roskam, I. (2019). Parental burnout: What is it, and why does it matter? *Clinical Psychological Science, 7*(6), 1319–1329. https://doi.org/10.1177/2167702619858430

Mills-Koonce, W. R., Propper, C., Gariepy, J. L., Barnett, M., Moore, G. A., Calkins, S., & Cox, M. J. (2009). Psychophysiological correlates of parenting behavior in mothers of young children. *Developmental Psychobiology, 51*(8), 650–661. https://doi.org/10.1002/dev.20400

Mills, P., Newman, E. F., Cossar, J., & Murray, G. (2015). Emotional maltreatment and disordered eating in adolescents: Testing the mediating role of emotion regulation. *Child Abuse & Neglect, 39*, 156–166. https://doi.org/10.1016/j.chiabu.2014.05.011

Mitchell, J. P. (2009). Social psychology as a natural kind. *Trends in Cognitive Sciences, 13*(6), 246–251. https://doi.org/10.1016/j.tics.2009.03.008

Mitsven, S., Messinger, D. S., Moffitt, J., & Ahn, Y. A. (2020). Infant emotional development. In J. J. Lockman & C. S. Tamis-LeMonda (Eds.), *The Cambridge handbook of infant development: Brain, behavior, and cultural context* (pp. 742–776). Cambridge University Press. https://doi.org/10.1017/9781108351959.027

Molenberghs, P., Johnson, H., Henry, J. D., & Mattingley, J. B. (2016). Understanding the minds of others: A neuroimaging meta-analysis. *Neuroscience and Biobehavioral Reviews, 65*, 276–291. https://doi.org/10.1016/j.neubiorev.2016.03.020

Monk, C., Spicer, J., & Champagne, F. A. (2012). Linking prenatal maternal adversity to developmental outcomes in infants: The role of epigenetic pathways. *Development and Psychopathology, 24*, 1361–1376. https://doi.org/10.1017/S0954579412000764

Morgan P. L., Farkas G., Hillemeier M. M., Hammer C. S., Maczuga S. (2015). 24-month-old children with larger oral vocabularies display greater academic and behavioral functioning at kindergarten entry. *Child Development, 86*, 1351–1370. https://doi.org/10.1111/cdev.12398

Morishima, Y., Schunk, D., Bruhin, A., Ruff, C. C., & Fehr, E. (2012). Linking brain structure and activation in temporoparietal junction to explain the neurobiology of human altruism. *Neuron, 75*(1), 73–79. https://doi.org/10.1016/j.neuron.2012.05.021

Morrison, I., Löken, L. S., & Olausson, H. (2010). The skin as a social organ. *Experimental Brain Research, 204*(3), 305–314. https://doi.org/10.1007/s00221-009-2007-y

Mosley P. E. (2009). Bigorexia: Bodybuilding and muscle dysmorphia. *European Eating Disorders Review: The Journal of the Eating Disorders Association, 17*(3), 191–198. https://doi.org/10.1002/erv.897

Moulson, M. C., Shutts, K., Fox, N. A., Zeanah, C. H., Spelke, E. S., & Nelson, C. A. (2015). Effects of early institutionalization on the development of emotion processing: A case for relative sparing? *Developmental Science, 18*(2), 298–313. https://doi.org/10.1111/desc.12217

Mountford, V., Corstorphine, E., Tomlinson, S., & Waller, G. (2007). Development of a measure to assess invalidating childhood environments in the eating disorders. *Eating Behaviors, 8*(1), 48–58. https://doi.org/10.1016/j.eatbeh.2006.01.003

Mphaphuli, L. K. (2023). The impact of dysfunctional families on the mental health of children. *IntechOpen.* https://doi.org/10.5772/intechopen.110565

Mullen, P. E., Martin, J. L., Anderson, J. C., Romans, S. E., & Herbison, G. P. (1996). The long-term impact of the physical, emotional, and sexual abuse of children: A community study. *Child Abuse & Neglect, 20*(1), 7–21. https://doi.org/10.1016/0145-2134(95)00112-3

Muscatell, K. A., Morelli, S. A., Falk, E. B., Way, B. M., Pfeifer, J. H., Galinsky, A. D., ... & Eisenberger, N. I. (2012). Social status modulates neural activity in the mentalizing network. *NeuroImage, 60*(3), 1771–1777. https://doi.org/10.1016/j.neuroimage.2012.01.080

Musetti, A., Cattivelli, R., Giacobbi, M., Zuglian, P., Ceccarini, M., Capelli, F., Pietrabissa, G., & Castelnuovo, G. (2016). Challenges in internet addiction disorder: Is a diagnosis feasible or not? *Frontiers in Psychology, 7*, 842. doi: 10.3389/fpsyg.2016.00842. PMID: 27375523; PMCID: PMC4894006.

Musetti, A., Grazia, V., Manari, T., Terrone, G., & Corsano, P. (2021). Linking childhood emotional neglect to adolescents' parent-related loneliness: Self-other differentiation and emotional detachment from parents as mediators. *Child Abuse & Neglect, 122*, 105338. https://doi.org/10.1016/j.chiabu.2021.105338

Myruski, S., Gulyayeva, O., Birk, S., Pérez-Edgar, K., Buss, K. A., & Dennis-Tiwary, T. A. (2018). Digital disruption? Maternal mobile device use is related to infant social-emotional functioning. *Developmental Science, 21*(4), e12610. https://doi.org/10.1111/desc.12610

Narvaez, D., Wang, L., Cheng, A., Gleason, T. R., Woodbury, R., Kurth, A., & Lefever, J. B. (2019). The importance of early life touch for psychosocial and moral development. *Psicologia, reflexao e critica: revista semestral do Departamento de Psicologia da UFRGS, 32*(1), 16. https://doi.org/10.1186/s41155-019-0129-0

Nathanson, A. I., & Rasmussen, E. E. (2011). TV viewing compared to book reading and toy playing reduces responsive maternal communication with toddlers and preschoolers. *Human Communication Research, 37*(4), 465–487. https://doi.org/10.1111/j.1468-2958.2011.01413.x

Naughton, A. M., Maguire, S. A., Mann, M. K., Lumb, R. C., Tempest, V., Gracias, S., & Kemp, A. M. (2013). Emotional, behavioral, and developmental features indicative of neglect or emotional abuse in preschool children: A systematic review. *JAMA Pediatrics, 167*(8), 769–775. https://doi.org/10.1001/jamapediatrics.2013.192

Nazlıgül, M. D., Yılmaz, A. E., & Griffiths, M. D. (2023). Gaming addiction and exercise addiction: To what extent are they the same or different in terms of emotional abuse and/or emotional neglect etiologies? *International Journal of Mental Health and Addiction, 21*, 145–164. https://doi.org/10.1007/s11469-021-00585-0

Neil, L., Viding, E., Armbruster-Genc, D., Lisi, M., Mareschal, I., Rankin, G., & McCrory, E. (2022). Trust and childhood maltreatment: Evidence of bias in appraisal of unfamiliar faces. *Journal of Child Psychology and Psychiatry, 63*(6), 655–662. https://doi.org/10.1111/jcpp.13503

Nemati, H., Sahebihagh, M. H., Mahmoodi, M., Ghiasi, A., Ebrahimi, H., Barzanjeh Atri, S., & Mohammadpoorasl, A. (2020). Non-suicidal self-injury and its relationship with family psychological function and perceived social support among

Iranian high school students. *Journal of Research in Health Sciences, 20*(1), e00469. https://doi.org/10.34172/jrhs.2020.04

Neumark-Sztainer, D., Paxton, S. J., Hannan, P. J., Haines, J., & Story, M. (2006). Does body satisfaction matter? Five-year longitudinal associations between body satisfaction and health behaviors in adolescent females and males. *The Journal of Adolescent Health: Official Publication of the Society for Adolescent Medicine, 39*(2), 244–251. https://doi.org/10.1016/j.jadohealth.2005.12.001

Nijenhuis, E. R. S., & van der Hart, O. (2011). Dissociation in trauma: A new definition and comparison with previous formulations. *Journal of Trauma & Dissociation, 12*(4), 416–445. https://doi.org/10.1080/15299732.2011.570592

Nikolakis, W., & Nelson, H. (2019). Trust, institutions, and indigenous self-governance: An exploratory study. *Governance, 32*(3), 331–347. https://doi.org/10.1111/gove.12374

Nolin, P., & Ethier, L. (2007). Using neuropsychological profiles to classify neglected children with or without physical abuse. *Child Abuse & Neglect, 31*(6), 631–643. https://doi.org/10.1016/j.chiabu.2006.12.009

Norman, R. E., Byambaa, M., De, R., Butchart, A., Scott, J., & Vos, T. (2012). The long-term health consequences of child physical abuse, emotional abuse, and neglect: A systematic review and meta-analysis. *PLoS Medicine, 9*(11), e1001349. https://doi.org/10.1371/journal.pmed.1001349

Nummenmaa, L., Hari, R., Hietanen, J. K., & Glerean, E. (2018). Maps of subjective feelings. *Proceedings of the National Academy of Sciences,* 115(37), 9198–9203. https://doi.org/10.1073/pnas.1807390115

O'Donnell, M. L., Lau, W., Chisholm, K., Agathos, J., Little, J., Terhaag, S., ... & Gallagher, M. W. (2021). A pilot study of the efficacy of the unified protocol for transdiagnostic treatment of emotional disorders in treating posttraumatic psychopathology: A randomized controlled trial. *Journal of Traumatic Stress, 34*(3), 563–574. https://doi.org/10.1002/jts.22650

Okoye, C., Obialo-Ibeawuchi, C. M., Obajeun, O. A., Sarwar, S., Tawfik, C., Waleed, M. S., ... & Mbaezue, R. N. (2023). Early diagnosis of autism spectrum disorder: A review and analysis of the risks and benefits. *Cureus, 15*(8), e43226. https://doi.org/10.7759/cureus.43226

Oláh, K., & Király, I. (2019). Young children selectively imitate models conforming to social norms. *Frontiers in Psychology, 10,* 1399. https://doi.org/10.3389/fpsyg.2019.01399

Oncioiu, S. I., Orri, M., Boivin, M., Geoffroy, M. C., Arseneault, L., Brendgen, M., ... & Côté, S. M. (2020). Early childhood factors associated with peer victimization trajectories from 6 to 17 years of age. *Pediatrics, 145*(5), 1–10. https://doi.org/10.1542/peds.2019-2654

Orben, A., Tomova, L., & Blakemore, S. J. (2020). The effects of social deprivation on adolescent development and mental health. *The Lancet Child & Adolescent Health, 4*(8), 634–640. https://doi.org/10.1016/S2352-4642(20)30186-3

Orsillo, S. M., Batten, S. V., Plumb, J. C., Luterek, J. A., & Roessner, B. M. (2004). An experimental study of emotional responding in women with posttraumatic stress disorder related to interpersonal violence. *Journal of Traumatic Stress, 17,* 241–248. https://doi.org/10.1023/B:JOTS.0000029267.61240.94

Osorio, A., Lopez-del Burgo, C., Carlos, S., & de Irala, J. (2017). The sooner, the worse? Association between earlier age of sexual initiation and worse adolescent health and well-being outcomes. *Frontiers in Psychology, 8*, 1298. https://doi.org/10.3389/fpsyg.2017.01298

Pan, H., & Zhang, Y. (2023). Understanding the emotional development of school-aged children: A critical review. *Journal of Education, Humanities and Social Sciences, 8*, 1860–1866. https://doi.org/10.54097/ehss.v8i.4597

Parham, L., & Primeau, L. (1997). Play and occupational therapy. In L. D. Parham & L. Fazio (Eds.), *Play in occupational therapy for children* (pp. 2–21). Mosby.

Paris, J. (2015). *Overdiagnosis in psychiatry*. Oxford University Press.

Paulus, M., Becher, T., Christner, N., Kammermeier, M., Gniewosz, B., & Pletti, C. (2024). When do children begin to care for others? The ontogenetic growth of empathic concern across the first two years of life. *Cognitive Development, 70*, 101439. https://doi.org/10.1016/j.cogdev.2024.101439

Pearce, E., Wlodarski, R., Machin, A., & Dunbar, R. I. M. (2017). Variation in the β-endorphin, oxytocin, and dopamine receptor genes is associated with different dimensions of human sociality. *Proceedings of the National Academy of Sciences, 114*(20), 5300–5305. https://doi.org/10.1073/pnas.1700712114

Peichl, J. (2007). *Innere Kinder, Täter, Helfer & Co: Ego-State-Therapie des traumatisierten Selbst*. Klett-Cotta.

Penner, F., Gambin, M., & Sharp, C. (2019). Childhood maltreatment and identity diffusion among inpatient adolescents: The role of reflective function. *Journal of Adolescence, 76*, 65–74. https://doi.org/10.1016/j.adolescence.2019.08.002

Pitula, C. E., Wenner, J. A., Gunnar, M. R., & Thomas, K. M. (2016). To trust or not to trust: Social decision-making in post-institutionalized, internationally adopted youth. *Developmental Science*. https://doi.org/10.1111/desc.12375

Pohar, R., & Argáez, C. (2017). *Acceptance and commitment therapy for post-traumatic stress disorder, anxiety, and depression: A review of clinical effectiveness*. Canadian Agency for Drugs and Technologies in Health.

Polansky, N. A., Chalmers, M. A., Buttenwieser, E., & Williams, D. P. (1981). *Damaged parents: An anatomy of child neglect*. University of Chicago Press.

Polzer, J. C., & Knabe, S. M. (2012). From desire to disease: Human papillomavirus (HPV) and the medicalization of nascent female sexuality. *The Journal of Sex Research, 49*(4), 344–352. https://doi.org/10.1080/00224499.2011.644598

Pope, C. G., Pope, H. G., Menard, W., Fay, C., Olivardia, R., & Phillips, K. A. (2005). Clinical features of muscle dysmorphia among males with body dysmorphic disorder. *Body Image, 2*(4), 395–400. https://doi.org/10.1016/j.bodyim.2005.09.001

Prior, M. K., & Quinn, A. S. (2010). The relationship between childhood emotional neglect and adult spirituality: An exploratory study. *Journal of Religion & Spirituality in Social Work: Social Thought, 29*(4), 277–299. https://doi.org/10.1080/15426432.2010.518816

Rademacher, A., Goagoses, N., Schmidt, S., Zumbach, J., & Koglin, U. (2021). Preschoolers' profiles of self-regulation, social-emotional and behavior skills and its prediction for a successful behavior adaptation during the transitional period from preschool to elementary school. *Early Education and Development, 17*(4), 1–15. https://doi.org/10.1080/10409289.2021.1958283

Radesky, J. S., Peacock-Chambers, E., Zuckerman, B., & Silverstein, M. (2016). Use of mobile technology to calm upset children: Associations with social-emotional development. *JAMA Pediatrics, 170*(4), 397–399. https://doi.org/10.1001/jamapediatrics.2015.4260

Rantalainen, K., Paavola-Ruotsalainen, L., Alakortes, J., Carter, A. S., Ebeling, H. E., & Kunnari, S. (2021). Early vocabulary development: Relationships with prelinguistic skills and early social-emotional/behavioral problems and competencies. *Infant Behavior and Development, 62,* 101525. https://doi.org/10.1016/j.infbeh.2020.101525

Raudaskoski, S., Mantere, E., & Valkonen, S. (2017). The influence of parental smartphone use, eye contact and 'bystander ignorance' on child development. In *Social and political science 2017* (pp. 173–184). https://doi.org/10.4337/97817853 66673.00021

Raufelder, D., Neumann, N., Domin, M., Lorenz, R. C., Gleich, T., Golde, S., ... & Hoferichter, F. (2021). Do belonging and social exclusion at school affect structural brain development during adolescence? *Child Development.* https://doi.org/10.1111/cdev.13613

Raver, C. C., Garner, P., & Smith-Donald, R. (2007). The roles of emotion regulation and emotion knowledge for children's academic readiness: Are the links causal? In B. Pianta, K. Snow, & M. Cox (Eds.), *Kindergarten transition and early school success* (pp. 121–148). Brookes Publishing.

Rebbe, R. (2018). What is neglect? State legal definitions in the United States. *Child Maltreatment, 23*(3), 303–315. https://doi.org/10.1177/1077559518767337

Rees, C. (2008). The influence of emotional neglect on development. *Journal of Paediatrics and Child Health, 18*(12), 527–534. https://doi.org/10.1016/j.paed.2008.09.003

Reilly, E. B., & Gunnar, M. R. (2019). Neglect, HPA axis reactivity, and development. *International Journal of Developmental Neuroscience: The Official Journal of the International Society for Developmental Neuroscience, 78,* 100–108. https://doi.org/10.1016/j.ijdevneu.2019.07.010

Reinders, A. A. T. S., & Veltman, D. J. (2021). Dissociative identity disorder: Out of the shadows at last? *British Journal of Psychiatry, 219*(2), 413–414. https://doi.org/10.1192/bjp.2020.168

Reupert, A. (2020). *Mental health and academic learning in schools: Approaches for facilitating the wellbeing of children and young people.* Routledge.

Reyome, N. D. (1993). A comparison of the school performance of sexually abused, neglected and non-maltreated children. *Child Study Journal, 23,* 17–38.

Reyome, N. D. (2010). Childhood emotional maltreatment and later intimate relationships: Themes from the empirical literature. *Journal of Aggression, Maltreatment & Trauma, 19*(3), 224–242. https://doi.org/10.1080/10926770903539664

Rideout, V. (2017). *The common-sense census: Media use by kids age zero to eight.* Common Sense Media.

Rigby, K. (2022). *Multiperspectivity on school bullying: One pair of eyes in not enough.* Routledge.

Rizk, M., Mattar, L., Kern, L., Berthoz, S., Duclos, J., Viltart, O., & Godart, N. (2020). Physical activity in eating disorders: A systematic review. *Nutrients, 12*(1), 183. https://doi.org/10.3390/nu12010183

Roediger, E., Stevens, B. A., & Brockman, R. (2018). *Contextual schema therapy: An integrative approach to personality disorders, emotional dysregulation, and interpersonal functioning.* New Harbinger Publications.

Roeser, R. W., Eccles, J. S., & Sameroff, A. J. (2000). School as a context of early adolescents' academic and social-emotional development: A summary of research findings. *The Elementary School Journal, 100,* 443–471. http://dx.doi. org/10.1086/499650

Rogol, A. D. (2020). Emotional deprivation in children: Growth faltering and *reversible* hypopituitarism. *Frontiers in Endocrinology, 11,* 596144. https://doi. org/10.3389/fendo.2020.596144

Roskam, I., Brianda, M. E., & Mikolajczak, M. (2018). A step forward in the conceptualization and measurement of parental burnout: The parental burnout assessment (PBA). *Frontiers in Psychology, 9,* 758. https://doi.org/10.3389/fpsyg.2018.00758

Roth, M. C., Humphreys, K. L., King, L. S., & Gotlib, I. H. (2018). Self-reported neglect, amygdala volume, and symptoms of anxiety in adolescent boys. *Child Abuse & Neglect, 80,* 80–89. https://doi.org/10.1016/j.chiabu.2018.03.016

Rotholz, D. A., Kinsman, A. M., Lacy, K. K., & Charles, J. (2017). Improving early identification and intervention for children at risk for autism spectrum disorder. *Pediatrics, 139*(2), e20161061. https://doi.org/10.1542/peds.2016-1061

Roy, S. C. (2008). 'Taking charge of your health': Discourses of responsibility in English-Canadian women's magazines. *Sociology of Health & Illness, 30*(3), 463–477. https://doi.org/10.1111/j.1467-9566.2007.01066.x

Rubin, K., Fein, G. G., & Vandenberg, B. (1983). Play. In P. H. Mussen (Ed.), *Handbook of child psychology* (4th ed., Vol. 4, pp. 693–774). Socialization, Personality, and Social Development. Wiley.

Rueger SY, Katz RL, Risser HJ, & Lovejoy MC (2011). Relations between parental affect and parenting behaviors: A meta-analytic review. *Parenting: Science and Practice, 11,* 1–33. https://doi.org/10.1080/15295192.2011.539503

Ruffman, T. (2023). Belief it or not: How children construct a theory of mind. *Child Development Perspectives, 17*(2), 106–112. https://doi.org/10.1111/cdep.12483

Russ, S. W. (2007). Pretend play: A resource for children who are coping with stress and managing anxiety. *NYS Psychologist, 19*(5), 13–17.

Ryan, R. M., & Deci, E. L. (2017). *Self-determination theory: Basic psychological needs in motivation, development, and wellness.* The Guilford Press. https://doi. org/10.1521/978.14625/28806

Ryan, R. M., & Deci, E. L. (2000). Self-determination theory and the facilitation of intrinsic motivation, social development, and well-being. *The American Psychologist, 55*(1), 68–78. https://doi.org/10.1037//0003-066x.55.1.68

Rye, N. (2008). Play therapy as a mental health intervention for children and adolescents. *Journal of Family Health Care, 18*(1), 17–19.

Saleem, S., Karamat, A., Zahra, S. T., Subhan, S., & Mahmood, Z. (2021). Mediating role of emotional neglect and self-injurious behaviors in the relationship between family satisfaction and depression. *The Family Journal.* https://doi. org/10.1177/10664807211000725

Salokangas, R. K. R., Schultze-Lutter, F., Schmidt, S. J., Pesonen, H., Luutonen, S., Patterson, P., Graf von Reventlow, H., Heinimaa, M., From, T., & Hietala, J. (2020). Childhood physical abuse and emotional neglect are specifically associated with adult mental disorders. *Journal of Mental Health (Abingdon, England), 29*(4), 376–384. https://doi.org/10.1080/09638237.2018.1521940

Santor, D. A., Messervey, D., & Kusumakar, V. (2000). Measuring peer pressure, popularity, and conformity in adolescent boys and girls: Predicting school performance, sexual attitudes, and substance abuse. *Journal of Youth and Adolescence, 29,* 163–182. https://doi.org/10.1023/A:1005152515264

Saunders, R., Jacobvitz, D., Zaccagnino, M., Beverung, L. M., & Hazen, N. (2011). Pathways to earned-security: The role of alternative support figures. *Attachment & Human Development, 13*(4), 403–420. https://doi.org/10.1080/14616734.2011. 584405

Scheeringa M. S. (2021). Reexamination of diathesis stress and neurotoxic stress theories: A qualitative review of pre-trauma neurobiology in relation to posttraumatic stress symptoms. *International Journal of Methods in Psychiatric Research, 30*(2), e1864. https://doi.org/10.1002/mpr.186

Schimmenti, A., Maganuco, N. R., La Marca, L., Di Dio, N., Gelsomino, E., & Gervasi, A. M. (2015). "Why do I feel so bad?" Childhood experiences of emotional neglect, negative affectivity, and adult psychiatric symptoms. *Mediterranean Journal of Social Sciences, 6*(6 S1), 259.

Schlumpf, Y. R., Nijenhuis, E. R. S., Klein, C., Jäncke, L., & Bachmann, S. (2019). Functional reorganization of neural networks involved in emotion regulation following trauma therapy for complex trauma disorders. *NeuroImage. Clinical, 23*, 101807. https://doi.org/10.1016/j.nicl.2019.101807

Schmälzle, R., Brook O'Donnell, M., Garcia, J. O., Cascio, C. N., Bayer, J., Bassett, D. S., Vettel, J. M., & Falk, E. B. (2017). Brain connectivity dynamics during social interaction reflect social network structure. *Proceedings of the National Academy of Sciences of the United States of America, 114*(20), 5153–5158. https://doi. org/10.1073/pnas.1616130114

Schultz, P. W., Nolan, J. M., Cialdini, R. B., Goldstein, N. J., & Griskovicius, V. (2007). The constructive, destructive, and reconstructive power of social norms. *Psychological Science, 18*(5), 429–434. https://doi.org/10.1111/j.1467-9280.2007.01917.x

Schwartz, B., & Ward, A. (2004). Doing better but feeling worse: The paradox of choice. In *Positive psychology in practice* (pp. 86–104). Retrieved from https:// works.swarthmore.edu/fac-psychology/221

Seligman, M. E. P. (1974). Depression and learned helplessness. In: R. J. Friedman, M. M. Katz (eds). *The psychology of depression: Contemporary theory and research* (pp. 83–113). Winston-Wiley.

Selman, R. L. (1981). The development of interpersonal competence: The role of understanding in conduct. *Developmental Review, 1*, 401–422.

Sengsavang, S., Willemsen, K., & Krettenauer, T. (2015). Why be moral? Children's explicit motives for prosocial-moral action. *Frontiers in Psychology, 6*, 552. https:// doi.org/10.3389/fpsyg.2015.00552

Sheng, X., Yang, M., Ge, M., Zhang, L., Huang, C., Cui, S., ... & Zhou, X. (2022). The relationship between Internet addiction and childhood trauma in adolescents: The mediating role of social support. *Frontiers in Psychology, 13*, 996086. https:// doi.org/10.3389/fpsyg.2022.996086

Sheridan, C. L., & Radmacher, S. A. (1998). Health psychology. A challenge for the biomedical health model. *Instytut Psychologii Zdrowia PTP.* [in Polish]

Shin, M., & Kemps, E. (2020). Media multitasking as an avoidance coping strategy against emotionally negative stimuli. *Anxiety, Stress, and Coping, 33*(4), 440–451. https://doi.org/10.1080/10615806.2020.1745194

Shipman, K., Edwards, A., Brown, A., Swisher, L., & Jennings, E. (2005). Managing emotion in a maltreating context: A pilot study examining child neglect. *Child Abuse & Neglect, 29*(9), 1015–1029. https://doi.org/10.1016/j.chiabu. 2005.01.006

Sikora, T., & Górnik-Durose, M. (2013). On the mentality of the contemporary human, its sources and manifestations. In M. Górnik-Durose (Ed.), *Contemporary culture and health* (pp. 15–50). GWP. [in Polish]

Silva, C. F., Silva, I., Rodrigues, A., Sá, L., Beirão, D., Rocha, P., & Santos, P. (2022). Young people awareness of sexually transmitted diseases and contraception: A Portuguese population-based cross-sectional study. *International Journal of Environmental Research and Public Health, 19*(21), 13933. https://doi.org/10.3390/ijerph192113933

Singh, L., Morgan, J. L., & Best, C. T. (2002). Infants' listening preferences: Baby talk or happy talk? *Infancy: The Official Journal of the International Society on Infant Studies, 3*(3), 365–394. https://doi.org/10.1207/S15327078IN0303_5

Singh, N. N. & Singh Joy, S. D. (2021). *Mindfulness-based interventions with children and adolescents: Research and practice.* Routledge.

Slack, K. S., Holl, J., Altenbernd, L., McDaniel, M., & Stevens, A. B. (2003). Improving the measurement of child neglect for survey research: Issues and recommendations. *Child Maltreatment, 8*(2), 98–111. https://doi.org/10.1177/1077559502250827

Słońska, Z., & Misiuna, M. (1993). *Health promotion. Dictionary of basic terms.* Warsaw. [in Polish]

Smetana, J. G. (1981). Preschool children's conceptions of moral and social rules. *Child Development, 52*(4), 1333–1336. https://doi.org/10.2307/1129527

Snyder, C. R., & Fromkin, H. L. (1977). Abnormality as a positive characteristic: The development and validation of a scale measuring need for uniqueness. *Journal of Abnormal Psychology, 86*(5), 518–527. https://doi.org/10.1037/0021-843X.86.5.518

Sorce, J. F., & Emde, R. N. (1981). Mother's presence is not enough: Effect of emotional availability on infant exploration. *Developmental Psychology, 17*(6), 737–745. https://doi.org/10.1037/0012-1649.17.6.737

Sousa, V., Silva, P. R., Romão, A. M., & Coelho, V. A. (2023). Can an universal school-based social emotional learning program reduce adolescents' social withdrawal and social anxiety? *Journal of Youth and Adolescence, 52*(11), 2404–2416. https://doi.org/10.1007/s10964-023-01840-4

Spengler, F. B., Schultz, J., Scheele, D., Essel, M., Maier, W., Heinrichs, M., & Hurlemann, R. (2017). Kinetics and dose dependency of intranasal oxytocin effects on amygdala reactivity. *Biological Psychiatry, 82*(12), 885–894. https://doi.org/10.1016/j.biopsych.2017.04.015

Spiegel, D., & Cardeña, E. (1991). Disintegrated experience: The dissociative disorders revisited. *Journal of Abnormal Psychology, 100*(3), 366–378. https://doi.org/10.1037/0021-843X.100.3.366

Spinelli, A., Buoncristiano, M., Kovacs, V. A., Yngve, A., Spiroski, I., Obreja, G., ... & Breda, J. (2019). Prevalence of severe obesity among primary school children in 21 European countries. *Obesity Facts, 12*(2), 244–258. https://doi.org/10.1159/000500436

Šramová, B. (2015). Marketing and media communications targeted to children as consumers. *Procedia - Social and Behavioral Sciences, 191*, 1522–1527. https://doi.org/10.1016/j.sbspro.2015.04.568

Sroufe, L. A., Egeland, B., Carlson, E., & Collins, W. A. (2005). Placing early attachment experiences in developmental context. In K. E. Grossmann, K. Grossmann, & E. Waters (Eds.), *The power of longitudinal attachment research: From infancy and childhood to adulthood* (pp. 48–70). Guilford.

Stake, R. E. (1997). A case study. In L. Korporowicz (Ed.), *Evaluation in education* (pp. XX-XX). Oficyna Naukowa Publishing House. [in Polish]

Steele, K. R., Townsend, M. L., & Grenyer, B. F. S. (2019). Parenting and personality disorder: An overview and meta-synthesis of systematic reviews. *PloS One, 14*(10), e0223038. https://doi.org/10.1371/journal.pone.0223038

Stoltenborgh, M., Bakermans-Kranenburg, M. J., & van Ijzendoorn, M. H. (2013). The neglect of child neglect: A meta-analytic review of the prevalence of neglect. *Social Psychiatry and Psychiatric Epidemiology, 48*(3), 345–355. https://doi.org/10.1007/s00127-012-0549-y

Stoltenborgh, M., Bakermans-Kranenburg, M. J., Alink, L. R. A., & van IJzendoorn, M. H. (2015). The prevalence of child maltreatment across the globe: Review of a series of meta-analyses. *Child Abuse Review, 24*(1), 37–50. https://doi.org/10.1002/car.2353

Strathearn, L., Fonagy, P., Amico, J., & Montague, P. R. (2009). Adult attachment predicts maternal brain and oxytocin response to infant cues. *Neuropsychopharmacology, 34*(13), 2655–2666. doi: 10.1038/npp.2009.103. Epub 2009 Aug 26. PMID: 19710635; PMCID: PMC3041266.

Su, Y., D'Arcy, C., & Meng, X. (2022). Intergenerational effect of maternal childhood maltreatment on next generation's vulnerability to psychopathology: A systematic review with meta-analysis. *Trauma, Violence, & Abuse, 23*(1), 152–162. https://doi.org/10.1177/1524838020933870

Sullivan, H. S. (1953). *The interpersonal theory of psychiatry.* W W Norton & Co.

Sun, L., Canevello, A., Lewis, K. A., Li, J., & Crocker, J. (2021). Childhood emotional maltreatment and romantic relationships: The role of compassionate goals. *Frontiers in Psychology, 12*, 723126. https://doi.org/10.3389/fpsyg.2021.723126

Surya, A., Retnawati, H., & Haryanto. (2023). Findings and implications of social emotional learning (SEL) in paternalistic culture in elementary schools: A systematic literature review. *Pegem Journal of Education and Instruction, 13*(3), 151–158.

Swartz, J. R., Weissman, D. G., Ferrer, E., Beard, S. J., Fassbender, C., Robins, R. W., Hastings, P. D., & Guyer, A. E. (2020). Reward-related brain activity prospectively predicts increases in alcohol use in adolescents. *Journal of the American Academy of Child and Adolescent Psychiatry, 59*(3), 391–400. https://doi.org/10.1016/j.jaac.2019.05.022

Talmon, A., Horovitz, M., Shabat, N., Haramati, O. S., & Ginzburg, K. (2019). "Neglected moms" - The implications of emotional neglect in childhood for the transition to motherhood. *Child Abuse & Neglect, 88*, 445–454. https://doi.org/10.1016/j.chiabu.2018.12.021

Taylor, J. L., Henninger, N. A., & Mailick, M. R. (2015). Longitudinal patterns of employment and postsecondary education for adults with autism and average-range IQ. *Autism: The International Journal of Research and Practice, 19*(7), 785–793. https://doi.org/10.1177/1362361315585643

Thomasius, R., Paschke, K., & Arnaud, N. (2022). Substance-use disorders in children and adolescents. *Deutsches Arzteblatt International, 119*(25), 440–450. https://doi.org/10.3238/arztebl.m2022.0122

Thornberry, T. P., Ireland, T. O., & Smith, C. A. (2001). The importance of timing: The varying impact of childhood and adolescent maltreatment on multiple problem outcomes. *Development and Psychopathology, 13*(4), 957–979. https://doi.org/10.1017/S0954579401004114

Tomasello, M. (2000). The social-pragmatic theory of word learning. *Pragmatics, 10*(4), 401–413. https://doi.org/10.1075/prag.10.4.01tom

Tomé, G., Matos, M., Simões, C., Diniz, J. A., & Camacho, I. (2012). How can peer group influence the behavior of adolescents: Explanatory model. *Global Journal of Health Science, 4*(2), 26–35. https://doi.org/10.5539/gjhs.v4n2p26

Tracy, J. L., & Robins, R. W. (2007). The self in self-conscious emotions: A cognitive appraisal approach. In J. L. Tracy, R. W. Robins, & J. P. Tangney (Eds.), *The self-conscious emotions: Theory and research* (pp. 3–20). The Guilford Press.

Tran-Chi, V.-L., Huynh, S. V., Nguyen, H. T., Giang, T.-V., & Luu-Thi, H.-T. (2023). The perception of implementing social-emotional learning in soft skills among Vietnamese high school students. *ASEAN Journal of Psychiatry, 24*, 1–12. https://doi.org/10.54615/2231-7805.47331

Trickett, P. T., Mennen, F. E., Kim, K., & Sang, J. (2009). Emotional abuse in a sample of multiply-maltreated, urban young adolescents: Issues of definition and identification. *Child Abuse & Neglect, 33*, 27–35. https://doi.org/10.1016/j.chiabu.2008.12.005

Triggle, D. J. (2007). Calcium channel antagonists: Clinical uses--past, present and future. *Biochemical Pharmacology, 74*(1), 1–9. doi: 10.1016/j.bcp.2007.01.016. Epub 2007 Jan 13. PMID: 17276408.

Turkle, S. (2011). *Alone together: Why we expect more from technology and less from each other*. Basic Books. [Audiobook]

Turner, H. A., Finkelhor, D., & Ormrod, R. (2006). The effect of lifetime victimization on the mental health of children and adolescents. *Social Science and Medicine, 62*, 13–27. https://doi.org/10.1016/j.socscimed.2005.05.030

Tusche, A., Böckler, A., Kanske, P., Trautwein, F. M., & Singer, T. (2016). Decoding the charitable brain: Empathy, perspective taking, and attention shifts differentially predict altruistic giving. *The Journal of Neuroscience: The Official Journal of the Society for Neuroscience, 36*(17), 4719–4732. https://doi.org/10.1523/JNEUROSCI.3392-15.2016

Twenge, J. M., & Campbell, W. K. (2018). Associations between screen time and lower psychological well-being among children and adolescents: Evidence from a population-based study. *Preventive Medicine Reports, 12*, 271–283. https://doi.org/10.1016/j.pmedr.2018.10.003

Valente, M., Renckens, S., Bunders-Aelen, J., & Syurina, E. V. (2022). The #orthorexia community on Instagram. *Eating and Weight Disorders: EWD, 27*(2), 473–482. https://doi.org/10.1007/s40519-021-01157-w

Valtolina, G. G., Polizzi, C., & Perricone, G. (2023). Improving the early assessment of child neglect signs - A new technique for professionals. *Pediatric Reports, 15*(2), 390–395. https://doi.org/10.3390/pediatric15020035

van Bakel, H., Bastiaansen, C., Hall, R., Schwabe, I., Verspeek, E., Gross, J. J., ... & Roskam, I. (2022). Parental burnout across the globe during the COVID-19 pandemic. *International Perspectives in Psychology: Research, Practice, Consultation, 11*(3), 141–152. https://doi.org/10.1027/2157-3891/a000050

van den Bergh, B. R., Mennes, M., Stevens, V., van der Meere, J., Börger, N., Stiers, P., Marcoen, A., & Lagae, L. (2006). ADHD deficit as measured in adolescent boys with a continuous performance task is related to antenatal maternal anxiety. *Pediatric Research, 59*(1), 78–82. https://doi.org/10.1203/01.pdr.0000191143.75673.52

Van der Hart O., Nijenhuis E. R. S., & Steele K. (2006). *The haunted self: Structural dissociation and the treatment of chronic traumatization*. Norton

Vanden Abeele, M. M. P. (2020). Digital Well-being as a dynamic construct. *Communication Theory*. https://doi.org/10.1093/ct/qtaa024.

Vanden Abeele, M. M. P., Hendrickson, A. T., Pollmann, M. M. H., & Ling, R. (2019). Phubbing behavior in conversations and its relation to perceived conversation intimacy and distraction: An exploratory observation study. *Computers in Human Behavior, 100*, 35–47. https://doi.org/10.1016/j.chb.2019.05.004

Vasiliu O. (2023). At the crossroads between eating disorders and body dysmorphic disorders-the case of bigorexia nervosa. *Brain Sciences, 13*(9), 1234. https://doi.org/10.3390/brainsci13091234

Veale, J. F., Peter, T., Travers, R., & Saewyc, E. M. (2017). Enacted stigma, mental health, and protective factors among transgender youth in Canada. *Transgender Health, 2*(1), 207–216. https://doi.org/10.1089/trgh.2017.0031

Vermetten, E., & Lanius, R. A. (2012). Biological and clinical framework for post-traumatic stress disorder. *Handbook of Clinical Neurology, 106*, 291–342. https://doi.org/10.1016/B978-0-444-52002-9.00018-8

Vermetten, E., & Spiegel, D. (2014). Trauma and dissociation: Implications for borderline personality disorder. *Current Psychiatry Reports, 16*(2), 434. https://doi.org/10.1007/s11920-013-0434-8

Vieira Martins, M., Karara, N., Dembiński, L., Jacot-Guillarmod, M., Mazur, A., Hadjipanayis, A., & Michaud, P. A. (2023). Adolescent pregnancy: An important issue for paediatricians and primary care providers-A position paper from the European academy of paediatrics. *Frontiers in Pediatrics, 11*, 1119500. https://doi.org/10.3389/fped.2023.1119500

Vignoles, V. L., Chryssochoou, X., & Breakwell, G. M. (2000). The distinctiveness principle: Identity, meaning, and the bounds of cultural relativity. *Personality and Social Psychology Review, 4*(4), 337–354. https://doi.org/10.1207/S15327957PSPR0404_4

Vignoles, V. L., Schwartz, S. J., & Luyckx, K. (2011). Introduction: Toward an integrative view of identity. In S. J. Schwartz, K. Luyckx, & V. L. Vignoles (Eds.), *Handbook of identity theory and research, Vol. 1: Structures and processes* (pp. 1–27). Springer.

Vivanti, G., Prior, M., Williams, K., & Dissanayake, C. (2014). Predictors of outcomes in autism early intervention: Why don't we know more? *Frontiers in Pediatrics, 2*, 58. https://doi.org/10.3389/fped.2014.00058

von Klitzing, K., Simoni, H., & Bürgin, D. (1999). Child development and early triadic relationships. *The International Journal of Psycho-Analysis, 80* (Pt 1), 71–89. https://doi.org/10.1516/0020757991598576

Wang, C., Berry, B., & Swearer, S. M. (2013). The critical role of school climate in effective bullying prevention. *Theory into Practice, 52*, 296–302. https://doi.org/10.1080/00405841.2013.829735

Wang, Q., & Zhao, J. (2023). Emotional maltreatment and left-behind adolescents' loneliness in rural China: The moderating role of peer acceptance. *Current Psychology, 42*, 21478–21488. https://doi.org/10.1007/s12144-022-03263-z

Wang, X., Lee, M. Y., & Quinn, C. R. (2023). Intergenerational transmission of trauma: Unpacking the effects of parental adverse childhood experiences. *Journal of Family Studies, 29*(4), 1687–1703. https://doi.org/10.1080/13229400.2022.2073903

Wark, M. J., Kruczek, T., & Boley, A. (2003). Emotional neglect and family structure: Impact on student functioning. *Child Abuse & Neglect, 27*(9), 1033–1043. https://doi.org/10.1016/s0145-2134(03)00162-5

Waters, E., Weinfield, N. S., & Hamilton, C. E. (2000). The stability of attachment security from infancy to adolescence and early adulthood: General discussion. *Child Development, 71*(3), 703–706. https://doi.org/10.1111/1467-8624.00179

Watson, R. J., Wheldon, C. W., & Puhl, R. M. (2020). Evidence of diverse identities in a large national sample of sexual and gender minority adolescents. *Journal of Research on Adolescence, 30*(3), 431–442. https://doi.org/10.1111/jora.12488

Wei, M., Russell, D. W., Mallinckrodt, B., & Vogel, D. L. (2007). The experiences in close relationship scale (ECR)-short form: Reliability, validity, and factor structure. *Journal of Personality Assessment, 88*(2), 187–204. https://doi.org/10.1080/00223890701268041

Weinstein, A., & Szabo, A. (2023). Exercise addiction: A narrative overview of research issues. *Dialogues in Clinical Neuroscience, 25*(1), 1–13. https://doi.org/10.1080/19585969.2023.2164841

Wesarg-Menzel, C., Ebbes, R., Hensums, M., Wagemaker, E., Zaharieva, M. S., Staaks, J. P. C., ... & Wiers, R. W. (2023). Development and socialization of self-regulation from infancy to adolescence: A meta-review differentiating between self-regulatory abilities, goals, and motivation. *Developmental Review, 69*, 101090. https://doi.org/10.1016/j.dr.2023.101090

Wessells, M., & Kostelny, K. (2021). Understanding and ending violence against children: A holistic approach. Peace and conflict: *Journal of Peace Psychology, 27*(1), 3–23. http://dx.doi.org/10.1037/pac0000475

White, S. H. (1996). The child's entry into the "age of reason." In A. J. Sameroff & M. M. Haith (Eds.), *The five to seven year shift: The age of reason and responsibility* (pp. 17–30). University of Chicago Press.

Wildschut, M., Swart, S., Langeland, W., Smit, J. H., & Draijer, N. (2020). An emotional neglect-personality disorder approach: Quantifying a dimensional transdiagnostic model of trauma-related and personality disorders. *Journal of Personality Disorders, 34*(2), 250–261. https://doi.org/10.1521/pedi_2019_33_381

Willard, S. L., & Shively, C. A. (2016). *Social status and the non-human primate brain.* In C. Shively, & M. Wilson (Eds.), *Social inequalities in health in nonhuman primates. Developments in primatology: Progress and prospects.* Springer. https://doi.org/10.1007/978-3-319-30872-2_6

Williams, A. (2003). Adolescents' relationships with parents. *Journal of Language and Social Psychology, 22*(1), 58–65. https://doi.org/10.1177/0261927X02250056

Williams, K. D. (2007). Ostracism: The kiss of social death. *Social and Personality Psychology Compass, 1*(1), 236–247. https:// doi.org/10.1111/j.1751-9004.2007.00004.x

Wilson, B. J. (2008). Media and children's aggression, fear, and altruism. *The Future of Children, 18*(1). https://doi.org/10.1353/foc.0.0005

Wilson, N., Kariisa, M., Seth, P., Smith, H., 4th, & Davis, N. L. (2020). Drug and opioid-involved overdose deaths - United States, 2017–2018. *Morbidity and Mortality Weekly Report, 69*(11), 290–297. https://doi.org/10.15585/mmwr.mm6911a4

Winders, S. J., Murphy, O., Looney, K., & O'Reilly, G. (2020). Self-compassion, trauma, and posttraumatic stress disorder: A systematic review. *Clinical Psychology & Psychotherapy, 27*(3), 300–329. https://doi.org/10.1002/cpp.2429

Wirga, M., DeBernardi, M., Wirga, A., & Maultsby, M. C. (2020). Maultsby's rational behavior therapy: Background, description, practical applications, and recent developments. *Journal of Rational-Emotive & Cognitive-Behavior Therapy, 38*(4), 399–423. https://doi.org/10.1007/s10942-020-00341-8

Witte, T. H., & Mulla, M. M. (2013). Social norms for intimate partner violence. *Violence and Victims, 28*(6), 959–967. https://doi.org/10.1891/0886-6708.vv-d-12-00153

Wojtyna, E. & Stawiarska, P. (2013). On the contemporary understanding of health. In M. Górnik-Durose (Ed.), *Contemporary culture and health* (pp. 51–76). GWP. [in Polish]

Wojtyna, E., Hyla, M., Hachuła, A. (2024). Pain of threatened self: Explicit and implicit self-esteem, cortisol responses to a social threat and pain perception. *Journal of Clinical Medicine, 13*(9), 2705. https://doi.org/10.3390/jcm13092705

Wojtyna, E., Pasek, M., Nowakowska, A., Goździalska, A., & Jochymek, M. (2023). Self at risk: Self-esteem and quality of life in cancer patients undergoing surgical treatment and experiencing bodily deformities. *Healthcare, 11*(15), 2203. https://doi.org/10.3390/healthcare11152203

Wolfers, L. N., Kitzmann, S., Sauer, S., & Sommer, N. (2020). Phone use while parenting: An observational study to assess the association of maternal sensitivity and smartphone use in a playground setting. *Computers in Human Behavior, 102*, 31–38. https://doi.org/10.1016/j.chb.2019.08.013

Woodward, L. J., & Fergusson, D. M. (2000). Childhood peer relationship problems and later risks of educational under-achievement and unemployment. *Journal of Child Psychology and Psychiatry, and Allied Disciplines, 41*(2), 191–201.

World Health Organization. (2019). *International statistical classification of diseases and related health problems* (11th ed.). https://icd.who.int/browse11/l-m/en#/http://id.who.int/icd/entity/1804127841

World Health Organization. (2024). *Adolescent pregnancy.* https://www.who.int/news-room/fact-sheets/detail/adolescent-pregnancy

Wright, M. (2018). Cyberbullying victimization through social networking sites and adjustment difficulties: The role of parental mediation. *Journal of the Association for Information Systems, 19*(2), Article 1. https://aisel.aisnet.org/jais/vol19/iss2/1

Wu, K., Wang, F., Wang, W., & Li, Y. (2022). Parents' education anxiety and children's academic burnout: The role of parental burnout and family function. *Frontiers in Psychology, 12*, 764824. https://doi.org/10.3389/fpsyg.2021.764824

Xie, J., Luo, Y., & Chen, Z. (2023). Relationship between Partner phubbing and parent-adolescent relationship quality: A family-based study. *International Journal of Environmental Research and Public Health, 20*(1), 304. https://doi.org/10.3390/ijerph20010304

Xiong, T., Milios, A., McGrath, P. J., & Kaltenbach, E. (2022). The influence of social support on posttraumatic stress symptoms among children and adolescents: A scoping review and meta-analysis. *European Journal of Psychotraumatology, 13*(1), 2011601. https://doi.org/10.1080/20008198.2021.2011601

Xu, L., Becker, B., & Kendrick, K. M. (2019). Oxytocin facilitates social learning by promoting conformity to trusted individuals. *Frontiers in Neuroscience, 13*, 56. https://doi.org/10.3389/fnins.2019.00056

Yadavaia, J. E., Hayes, S. C., & Vilardaga, R. (2014). Using acceptance and commitment therapy to increase self-compassion: A randomized controlled trial.

Journal of Contextual Behavioral Science, 3(4), 248–257. https://doi.org/10.1016/j.jcbs.2014.09.002

Yaghoubi-Doust, M. (2013). Reviewing the association between the history of parental substance abuse and the rate of child abuse. *Addiction & Health, 5*(3–4), 126–133.

Yarkovsky, N., & Timmons Fritz, P. A. (2014). Attachment style, early sexual intercourse, and dating aggression victimization. *Journal of Interpersonal Violence, 29*(2), 279–298. https://doi.org/10.1177/0886260513505143

Ylitervo, L., Veijola, J., & Halt, A. H. (2023). Emotional neglect and parents' adverse childhood events. *European Psychiatry, 66*(1), e47. https://doi.org/10.1192/j.eurpsy.2023.2420

Yoshida, M., Takayanagi, Y., Inoue, K., Kimura, T., Young, L. J., Onaka, T., & Nishimori, K. (2009). Evidence that oxytocin exerts anxiolytic effects via oxytocin receptor expressed in serotonergic neurons in mice. *The Journal of Neuroscience: The Official Journal of the Society for Neuroscience, 29*(7), 2259–2271. https://doi.org/10.1523/JNEUROSCI.5593-08.2009

Young, H., Burke, L., & Nic Gabhainn, S. (2018). Sexual intercourse, age of initiation and contraception among adolescents in Ireland: Findings from the Health Behaviour in School-aged Children (HBSC) Ireland study. *BMC Public Health, 18*(1), 362. https://doi.org/10.1186/s12889-018-5217-z

Young, J. E., Klosko, J. S., & Weishaar, M. E. (2003). *Schema therapy: A practitioner's guide.* Guilford Press.

Young, R., Lennie, S., & Minnis, H. (2011). Children's perceptions of parental emotional neglect and control and psychopathology. *Journal of Child Psychology and Psychiatry, and Allied Disciplines, 52*(8), 889–897. https://doi.org/10.1111/j.1469-7610.2011.02390.x

Youngblade, L. M., & Belsky, J. (1988). Social and emotional consequences of child maltreatment. In R. Ammerman & M. Heusen (Eds.). *Children at risk: An evaluation of factors contributing to child abuse and neglect* (pp. 109–146). New Yo&Plenum.

Yu, S., &Liu, Q. X. (2020). Self-esteem and hope as mediators in the relationship of parental neglect to adolescents' suicide ideation. *Psychological Development and Education, 36*(3), 350–358

Zaccagnino, M., Cussino, M., Saunders, R., Jacobvitz, D., & Veglia, F. (2014). Alternative caregiving figures and their role on adult attachment representations. *Clinical Psychology & Psychotherapy, 21*(3), 276–287. https://doi.org/10.1002/cpp.1828

Zak, P. J., Kurzban, R., & Matzner, W. T. (2005). Oxytocin is associated with human trustworthiness. *Hormones and Behavior, 48*(5), 522–527. doi: 10.1016/j.yhbeh.2005.07.009. Epub 2005 Aug 18. PMID: 16109416.

Zaki, J., & Ochsner, K. N. (2012). The neuroscience of empathy: Progress, pitfalls and promise. *Nature Neuroscience, 15*(5), 675–680. https://doi.org/10.1038/nn.3085

Zauche, L. H., Thul, T. A., Mahoney, A. E. D., & Stapel-Wax, J. L. (2016). Influence of language nutrition on children's language and cognitive development: An integrated review. *Early Childhood Research Quarterly, 36*, 318–333. https://doi.org/10.1016/j.ecresq.2016.01.015

Zerubavel, N., Bearman, P. S., Weber, J., & Ochsner, K. N. (2015). Neural mechanisms tracking popularity in real-world social networks. *Proceedings of the*

National Academy of Sciences of the United States of America, 112(49), 15072–15077. https://doi.org/10.1073/pnas.1511477112

Zhang, D., Lee, E. K. P., Mak, E. C. W., Ho, C. Y., & Wong, S. Y. S. (2021). Mindfulness-based interventions: An overall review. *British Medical Bulletin, 138*(1), 41–57. https://doi.org/10.1093/bmb/ldab005

Zhang, Y., & Zhang, L. (2023). Relationship among aggression, non-suicidal self-injury, and depression in youths. *Iranian Journal of Public Health, 52*(8), 1711–1719. https://doi.org/10.18502/ijph.v52i8.13410

Zhang, Y., Zhan, N., Long, M., Xie, D., & Geng, F. (2022). Associations of childhood neglect, difficulties in emotion regulation, and psychological distresses to COVID-19 pandemic: An intergenerational analysis. *Child Abuse & Neglect, 129*, 105674. https://doi.org/10.1016/j.chiabu.2022.105674

Zhao, J., Guo, Z., Shi, H., Yu, M., Jiao, L., & Xu, Y. (2023). The relationship between parental phubbing and interpersonal aggression in adolescents: The role of rejection sensitivity and school climate. *Journal of Interpersonal Violence, 38*(11–12), 7630–7655. https://doi.org/10.1177/08862605221145722

Zhao, J., Sun, X., & Wang, Q. (2021). Emotional neglect and depressive symptoms of left-behind adolescents: The role of friendship quality and gender. *Journal of Affective Disorders, 295*, 377–383. https://doi.org/10.1016/j.jad.2021.08.073

Zheng, H., Bornman, J., Granlund, M., Zhao, Y., & Huus, K. (2023). Participation of children with long-term health conditions compared to that of healthy peers: A cross-sectional comparative study. *Scandinavian Journal of Occupational Therapy, 30*(3), 334–343. https://doi.org/10.1080/11038128.2022.2035815

Zins, J. E., & Elias, M. J. (2006). Social and emotional learning. In G. G. Bear & K. M. Minke (Eds.), *Children's needs III: Development, prevention, and intervention* (pp. 1–13). National Association of School Psychologists.

Zorn, P., Roder, V., Soravia, L., & Tschacher, W. (2008). Evaluation of the "Schema-focused emotive behavioural therapy" (SET) for patients with personality disorders: Results of a randomised controlled trial. *Psychother Psychosom Med Psychol, 58*, 371–378.

Zoromba, M. A., Abdelgawad, D., Hashem, S., El-Gazar, H., & Abd El Aziz, M. A. (2023). Association between media exposure and behavioral problems among preschool children. *Frontiers in Psychology, 14*, 1080550. https://doi.org/10.3389/fpsyg.2023.1080550

Zou, L. Q., Yang, Z. Y., Wang, Y., Lui, S. S., Chen, A. T., Cheung, E. F., & Chan, R. C. (2016). What does the nose know? Olfactory function predicts social network size in human. *Scientific Reports, 6*, 25026. https://doi.org/10.1038/srep25026

The proofreading of this book was co-financed by the funds granted under the Research Excellence Initiative of the University of Silesia in Katowice.

Index

Note: **Bold** page numbers refer to tables; *italic* page numbers refer to figures and page numbers followed by "n" denote endnotes.